The ADHD Affected Athlete

Michael E. Stabeno

Note for Librarians: a cataloguing record for this book that includes Dewey Classification and US Library of Congress numbers is available from the National Library of Canada. The complete cataloguing record can be obtained from the National Library's online database at:
www.nlc-bnc.ca/amicus/index-e.html

ISBN 1-4120-3242-3

TRAFFORD

This book was published on-demand in cooperation with Trafford Publishing.
On-demand publishing is a unique process and service of making a book available for retail sale to the public taking advantage of on-demand manufacturing and Internet marketing. On-demand publishing includes promotions, retail sales, manufacturing, order fulfilment, accounting and collecting royalties on behalf of the author.

Suite 6E, 2333 Government St., Victoria, B.C. V8T 4P4, CANADA
Phone   250-383-6864   Toll-free 1-888-232-4444 (Canada & US)
Fax   250-383-6804   E-mail   sales@trafford.com
Web site www.trafford.com   TRAFFORD PUBLISHING IS A DIVISION OF TRAFFORD HOLDINGS LTD.
Trafford Catalogue #04-1069   www.trafford.com/robots/04-1069.html
10   9   8   7   6   5   4   3

Dedicated to...

Liam, Brendan and every ADDer who ever got stuck in right field for not paying attention; or had to race against that stupid tortoise.

Special Thanks

I don't think it is possible to recognize or thank all the coaches, teachers and athletes who contributed to this book. I would like to recognize several people who made it possible.

Dr. David Conant-Norville, M.D. who graciously acted as my guide through the many medical issues involved in this subject.

Thanks to "The Wild Bunch" for showing me what ADDers could do if they were encouraged.

Thanks to Dave Elligott who was the first coach to apply what is in the book.

Thanks to "Pokey" Allen, Bert Allinger, Lorne Davies, Mike Jones, Roy Pitmon, Rob Baarts, and Clive Charles; all of whom encouraged every athlete to develop the gifts they were born with.

Thanks to my wife Karen for her encouragement and motivation..."Write the damn book because no one else is going to."

Table of Contents

Foreword

Finally!

We now have a guide to understanding and coaching the athlete with Attention Deficit Hyperactivity Disorder (ADHD). ADHD is a common psychiatric disorder that affects between 6-8% of children. Symptoms often persist into adulthood; therefore, athletes with this disorder are affected throughout their lifecycle. Many studies done over the last 20 years have validated ADHD's authenticity as a disorder and verified the effectiveness of treatment. Many books have been written for clinicians, and a handful of good books on ADHD have been authored for parents and educators. But until now, no information source on ADHD for athletic coaches has been available.

Quality coaching is one of the most important determinants affecting whether an athlete's sporting experience is successful, meaningful and rewarding. The responsibility of the coach is not only to instruct athletes in the skill and strategy necessary to compete, but also to create a positive experience for the athlete. Athletes who have fun and develop a vision of improvement will work hard in their sport and have a great chance of success. However, those athletes who become demoralized and discouraged eventually quit the sport to find some activity in which they feel more competent and successful. Hence, it is imperative for the coaches to learn as much as possible about strategies to help athletes turn weaknesses into strengths. The professional coach has the luxury of conferring with expert consultants regarding physical and psychological problems that may affect their athletes. Even some collegiate athletic departments have employed consulting sport psychiatrists for their athletes and coaches.

Unfortunately, coaches in youth sports rarely receive coaching training or instruction in normal child development, let alone some training in common medical, orthopedic and psychiatric problems. Informational and practical books like this one are important tools for coaches. In this book, Mike Stabeno effectively addresses common challenges faced by coaches of children, adolescents, and even adults affected by ADHD. His insights and recommendations are directed to coaches, but are equally relevant to teachers, employers and family members. Mike's personal experiences as an ADHD affected athlete, coach, and parent of two ADHD affected athletes, as well as his professional experience as a human resources manager, have equipped him well to write a book filled with practical information and usable coaching tips. Mike personalizes this book with his own experiences to illustrate his points.

As a child and adolescent psychiatrist with a long interest in youth sports, I see too often the pain that arises when an ADHD affected child or adolescent is coached by someone who does not understand the athlete or his/her disorder. The coach frequently becomes very frustrated with what are perceived to be the athlete's weaknesses and may overlook the athlete's unique strengths. These coaches are usually well- meaning individuals, but lack understanding and sensitivity to the needs of their athletes. This book dispels myths about ADHD and gives coaches a workable strategy to help give the ADHD affected athlete a chance to experience athletic success. Hopefully, with greater awareness about ADHD, the coach and athlete will work together more effectively, leading to more enjoyment for both.

David O. Conant-Norville M.D.[1]
Assistant Clinical Professor of Psychiatry
Oregon Health and Sciences University

---

[1] Dr. Conant-Norville is also a member of The International Society for Sport Psychiatry and founder of Mind Matters Clinic in Beaverton, Oregon.

Introduction

Why would a coach be interested in working with an ADHD affected athlete? The numbers indicate many already are and simply do not know it.

Each morning in America some six million students who have been diagnosed with ADHD receive medication so they can function "normally"[i]. How many high level athletes exist in a population of six million?

The percentage of the general population with ADHD is conservatively estimated at 6%, with three times as many men being diagnosed than women are.[ii] 6% of 280 million Americans is nearly seventeen million people. How many elite athletes would be found in a population of seventeen million?

So if you coach a soccer, softball, basketball, or baseball team, the odds are good that at least one of your players has ADHD.

If you are lucky, you will have more.

To understand why I make that statement it is critical that you understand how the athlete is affected by this condition. And this is more than the athlete being distractible, impulsive and hyperactive. It is how today's American society reacts to the ADDer[2].

For example, few people understand that the primary injury to the ADHD affected isn't caused by the condition, but by society's response to it. To constantly be told these behaviors are "wrong" and will not be tolerated is society's first attack on ADDers.

In the last twenty-five years life has become more difficult for the ADHD affected, particularly the ADHD affected athlete. I know this because I have ADHD and both my sons have ADHD.

During this period, American society has increasingly endorsed the adoption of group processes, consensus building, verbal communication, confrontation avoidance, conformity, neatness, and perfection.

But this endorsement censures ADHD's defining behaviors of distractibility, impulsivity and hyperactivity. And whether an organization, school or enterprise is a public or private entity it likely has a "zero tolerance" policy for anyone displaying what could be

---

2 For brevity I use the term ADDer when referring to anyone who has been diagnosed with ADHD, with or without hyperactivity.

interpreted as aggressive, confrontational, argumentative, or "inappropriate" activity.

Unarguably, the words distractible, impulsive and hyperactive have negative connotations. Subsequently every discussion about ADHD automatically starts with the unquestioned assumption these three behaviors are wrong and must be prevented or eliminated.

But are they wrong or are they just mislabeled? What if synonyms with positive connotations are substituted for distractible, impulsive and hyperactive?

Someone who is easily distracted by what goes on around them can also be described as being aware of their surroundings. The opposite of being aware is being unaware.

Another word for impulsive is spontaneous. And the opposite of spontaneous is cautious.

Another word for hyperactive is energetic. The opposite of energetic is lethargic.

If you coach a sports team do you want players who are unaware, cautious and lethargic? Or would you want players to be aware, spontaneous and energetic?

As stated earlier, if you are lucky, you will have more than one ADDer on your team.

"The Wild Bunch"

Our oldest son, Liam, was diagnosed with ADHD in the 4th grade. About this same time I received a phone call asking if I would be interested in coaching his AAU/YMCA basketball team. Since I had never played organized basketball (I wrestled and played football through high school and university) my immediate thought was I didn't know enough about the sport to coach it. When I shared this with the AAU/YMCA I was told not to worry. Basically my job was to be the adult and that the team needed a coach immediately because the season was starting the next week and the person who had been slated to coach had just been transferred. I agreed to coach if they didn't find anyone else. I suspect they immediately filled my name in as "Coach" and stopped looking.

Sometime during the first few practices three parents made the opportunity to speak with me privately. After some small talk about how much they appreciated me coaching their son, and how much he was looking forward to playing basketball, each conversation went something like this.

"Mike, I wanted to ask you to keep an eye on my son. He might seem a little off-task and impulsive every now and then."

"Off task? Impulsive?"

"Well, he has ADHD and his medication might be wearing off during practice. He might seem just a little ummm, ahhhh, well distracted and impulsive. But it really shouldn't be a problem."

Yeah, right.

The first few practices were disasters.

While I tried to share my rules, world view, philosophies, and values with the team "they" were constantly bouncing or kicking basketballs, poking one another, talking and generally not paying any attention to me, their coach. As to running any of the intricately choreographed plays, I might as well have been telling the tide to go out.

One of the fallouts of being the last team with a coach was receiving the last pick of colors for game "t-shirts". Our color was, for a group of nine-year old boys, a decidedly unpopular pink. After doing my very best to spin this "girl color" into a rugged, outdoorsy Pacific Northwest "guy color" of "Steelhead Red", one of "them" blurted out the obvious reality. *"But coach, it's still pink!"*

I was "stuck" with two teams. I had a group of small "John Stocktons"; attentive, respectful, obedient and "coachable". They loved practicing free throws and running set plays. They were right out of the casting call from "Little House on the Prairie" or "Leave it to Beaver" (sans Eddie Haskel).

And then there was "The Wild Bunch"; inattentive, rude, impulsive, disobedient, loudly outspoken and completely reactive. They hated practicing free throws and set plays. Individually they reminded me of Dennis Rodman and Robin Williams.

I couldn't believe that the YMCA had saddled me with a group of kids who couldn't keep a thought in their head long enough to finish tying their shoe. How on earth was I going to be able to win any basketball games with this group? It just wasn't fair to me, their coach.

And the league rules only increased my frustrations. Each player was guaranteed to play at least half the game. With ten players that meant everyone played half the game; period. I couldn't keep the "Wild Bunch" on the bench, only playing them a few token moments at the end of the game.

My first solution was to split the team into two equal "platoons", each with two of the "Wild

Bunch." My thought was to run the offense through the three other players, until "they" learned the plays.

The team lost its first game badly. No one seemed to have had any fun and there was a great deal of bickering going on. While the specifics are likely best forgotten, I do remember one comment from that game. After I asked one of "them" why he had flung a pass behind a teammate and out of bounds he responded *"Coach he was open, he just didn't know it."*

This wasn't going at all as I felt it should or the way I had been coached as I was growing up.

It is funny how fate plays a role in our lives. One of the many rules I handed out at the first practice was that you didn't start if you were late for practice. Surprisingly the "Wild Bunch" were all on time for the two practices before our second game. So when I announced the same starting line up for the second game the "Wild Bunch" immediately and loudly reminded me of my rule.

Could they have been listening?

I glanced at the other team perfectly running a weave drill for warm-ups. They wore matching black t-shirts, shorts, socks and Air Jordan's (discounted for their coach who worked at Nike). I looked across the court to where my wife sat in a chair. She immediately glanced down at her shoes.

I was caught by my own rules.[3]

Hoping we wouldn't fall too far behind, I soberly cautioned them to slow the game down, to play in control, run the set offense, and not to make any mistakes. "They" bounced basketballs, poked one another and generally ignored me. One had stuffed some cotton up his nose to stop the bleeding from where his sister had punched him during their car ride to the game. Another mentioned he didn't remember the plays. But his best friend (our "Point Guard") said that was okay because he didn't remember them either.

I was suddenly overwhelmed by the realization I had no control over this bunch of 4th graders. Nothing I could say would change the fact "they" were going to do exactly what they wanted to on the court. Stunned by this insight, I surrendered. I simply told "them" to play as hard and as fast as they could, fight for every rebound and loose ball. It didn't matter

---

[3] In retrospect I now realize that since each player was on the court for half the game, this particular rule was pointless. I adopted it simply because it was one I had followed during my playing days.

as long as they played hard. Suddenly "they" became still, warily eyeing me as if I had stepped off a spaceship.

"Coach, we'll get in trouble, we'll foul out."

I assured them as long as they played as hard as they could they wouldn't be in any trouble. *"Guys, they give you five fouls for a reason. You're supposed to use some of them. Just don't think about it."* I sent them onto the floor with that instruction. *"Just play, don't think about it!"*

Have you ever thrown breadcrumbs to ducks at a pond?

They played like ducks fighting for pieces of bread at the pond. They squawked, lunged, flapped their arms, threw themselves after every loose (or semi-loose) ball and rebound. They blocked shots, intercepted passes, took charges, and as they were falling out of bounds tapped balls in to team mates. At the end of the first quarter they were ahead 16-0, mostly on lay ups off turnovers.

I saw the other coach yelling at the same two teenaged referees I had yelled at the week before. And then telling the other team to *"Slow the game down"*, *"Control the ball"*, *"Run the set offense"*, and my favorite, *"Don't make any mistakes."*

And the Wild Bunch were all talking, laughing, and poking one another, not paying any attention to me or anyone else. But they were having fun doing exactly what each was born to do, go through life with the accelerator all the way to the floor.

And I experienced an epiphany.

Coaching ADHD affected athletes wasn't about perfection, planned plays or control; it was about speed, simplicity, and freedom. It was about them playing a style that suited their strengths, not someone else's strengths. For them it was about throwing gallons of paint on the wall, not trying to fill in a "paint by number" watercolor of what someone else had created.

And whether I gave them permission to or not they wanted to play the game on the ragged edge of chaos. But it was so much more fun for them to have permission.

And in the end, having fun was what it was all about for them.

Or, as one of my colleagues used to say, "Well duh!"

What Is ADHD?

Attention Deficit Hyperactivity Disorder (ADHD) seems to be fodder for talk radio, television, books, newspapers, magazines, barbershops, teacher lunch rooms, internet chat rooms, coffee shops, self help groups, and countless studies and reports. The condition directly affects teachers, school counselors, administrators, medical practitioners, psychologists, psychiatrists, employers, attorneys, judges and parents. Because of this interest, information is readily available on identification, diagnosis, behavior modification, medical treatment, medications, classroom teaching techniques, workplace layout, legal rights & obligations, reasonable accommodation, discipline, and a myriad of other issues.

But there is almost nothing dealing with the ADHD affected athlete.

What information that is available warns of supposed risks rather than the actual benefits of ADHD affected athletes; "Beware, ADHD Affected Athletes." A present day corollary to the "hic sunt dracones!" (Here There Are Dragons!) written on medieval charts to warn mariners of dragons lying in wait for the unwary.

This book then is written to provide athletic coaches with an insight into the condition and how it affects athletes and others. It provides some guidelines and techniques to better address the challenges and rewards of coaching ADHD affected athletes.

It is also intended to provide the parents of ADHD affected athletes with some awareness to the challenges and rewards of athletics for their son or daughter.

It represents no new scientific data on the condition, nor commentary on the social implications of ADHD. People far better educated and qualified than I routinely address these issues in other forums.

But before going any further into this subject, it is essential to establish what ADHD is, and what it is not.

First, the term Attention Deficit Hyperactivity Disorder is a misnomer. Since ADDers pay attention to everything, we don't have an attention deficit. We have a problem in filtering out what is going on. We are distracted by, or notice, almost everything.

ADHD is a long recognized[iii] chronic human condition represented in varying degrees by short attention span, distractibility, impulsivity, disorganization, hyperactivity and stimulation seeking.

People with ADHD are easily distracted, impulsive, and highly reactive to their environment. They tend to be disorganized, have difficulty planning, executing and finishing tasks (particularly those involving sequential steps). ADDers have difficulty comprehending only verbal instructions, and are often unacceptably active in settings such as a classroom, a meeting room or a gym. texting better

Also, the severity of the condition is different for each affected person. Some diagnoses result in no medication and little in the way of classroom accommodations. Other diagnoses will result in significant prescription medication, accommodations and behavior modifications. It is reasonable to surmise that many cases can be undiagnosed for years, maybe never being diagnosed.

I suspect at one time or another everyone has displayed most of these behaviors. But where unaffected people can readily control their behaviors, for the ADHD affected individual such a choice is not an option. Confronting these tendencies is an every day, all day struggle for the ADDer.

Diagnosing ADHD

ADHD is not an easily diagnosed condition such as diabetes, blindness, deafness or a physical deformity. Nonetheless given the condition's century old medical observation the popularly held belief that the condition is somehow a recent creation of child psychologists, quack doctors, drug companies and public school educators, simply doesn't hold up to scrutiny.

No definitive test or physical examination presently exists (such as for diabetes) to confirm the existence of ADHD. Rather trained medical professionals using an extensive array of tools perform a clinical diagnosis. These tools include multiple interviews, personal observations, tests and reviewing the individual's personal history (such as school performance, employment history, family relations, etc.).

Typically this process begins after the individual has begun school and these behaviors become apparent in comparison to others. This diagnosis occurs by observing or confirming student distractibility during class, and the inability to finish schoolwork assignments. Impulsivity often takes the form of speaking and acting out of turn, taking things away from other children, picking fights, etc. The diagnosis can take several weeks to complete.

According to National Institute for Mental Health (NIMH), medical professionals who may diagnose ADHD are psychiatrists, psychologists, pediatricians/family physicians, and neurologists.[iv]

Someone who is not a medical doctor or similarly trained professional should never attempt to diagnose or even suggest someone suffers from ADHD. If you are asked your opinion, bite your tongue and suggest that if the questioner, usually a parent, feels strongly enough to ask you the question, he or she might want to talk with a medical doctor, school counselor, or other qualified professional about it.

I would hope any coach would willingly volunteer whatever assistance possible to that process. If you are involved in a school setting, you might want to discuss your personal observations of the individual with appropriate staff members such as counselors, administrators or other school district personnel.

Contributing to the difficulty in diagnosing ADHD is it often occurs with other learning disabilities. These may include dyslexia, depression, Tourette's syndrome, and obsessive-compulsive behavior among others.

To aid in diagnosing the condition health professionals utilize the following list of symptoms from the Diagnosis and Statistical Manual-IV (DSM-IV). [v]

DSM-IV creates two distinctive clusters of ADHD behaviors: ADHD with a hyperactivity-impulsivity component and without a hyperactivity-impulsivity component. Some have argued sufficient hyperactivity-impulsivity components alone represent a subtype of ADHD. But as a layman I find the logic of this argument suspect. Since by definition ADHD is an attentional disorder, how can it be present without some form of "attentional deficit"?

Distractibility arrives from two sources. These are the external events of the surrounding environment such as birds flying, people talking and walking, cars driving by, radios playing, sunny weather, or anything else that occurs.

The other source of distractions is internal or the ADDer mind. Our thoughts, fears and memories seem to have a passkey into our consciousness. Irrespective of how hard we try to ignore them, like a group of uninvited houseguests they unlock the door and barge into our consciousness.

But the bigger problem caused by distractions from either sources is once they do take their leave; it is time consuming to remember what we were concentrating on before they barged in.

The reader should keep in mind the following diagnostic criterion is provided here only for illustrative purpose. Only qualified medical professionals should ever even attempt to make a diagnosis. Nor should the reader consider any of the information in this book to be professional medical advice. Always check with medical professionals for guidance on medical issues.

Inattention Behaviors

Six or more of the following symptoms of inattention have persisted for at least six months to a degree that is maladaptive and inconsistent with developmental level:

Often fails to give close attention to details or makes careless mistakes in schoolwork, work or other activities.

Often has difficulty sustaining attention in tasks or play activities.

Often does not seem to listen when spoken to directly.

Often does not follow through on instructions and fails to finish schoolwork, chores, or duties in the workplace.

Often has difficulty organizing tasks and activities.

Often avoids, dislikes or is reluctant to engage in tasks that require sustained mental effort (such as schoolwork or homework).

Often loses things necessary for tasks or activities (toys, assignments, pencils, books or tools).

Is often easily distracted by extraneous stimuli.

Is often forgetful in daily activities.

Hyperactivity-Impulsivity Behaviors

Six or more of the following symptoms of hyperactivity-impulsivity have persisted for at least six months to a degree that is maladaptive and inconsistent with developmental level:

Often blurts out answers before questions have been completed.

Often has difficulty waiting turn.

Often interrupts or intrudes on others, (e.g. butts into conversations or games).

Often fidgets with hands or feet or squirms in seat.

Often leaves seat in classroom or in other situations in which remaining seated is expected.

Often runs about or climbs incessantly in situations where it is inappropriate.

Often has difficulty playing or engaging in leisure activities quietly.

Is often "on the go" or acts as if "driven by a motor".

Often talks incessantly.

What Causes ADHD?

One of the first questions asked when someone is first confronted by ADHD is "Where did it come from?" Is ADHD caused by diet, the school system, religion, day care, television and video game violence or lack of exercise? Is it a learned behavior, or is it simply a fashionable excuse for being lazy or defiant?

First, the condition tends to run in families, with a strong tendency to be passed from one generation to the next. For example I have ADHD, as do both of my sons.

Research has also established a strong genetic component to the condition and current research is focusing on specific human genes.[vi]

So one day we might be able to determine the existence of, or likelihood of someone developing ADHD, with a simple blood test rather than the current lengthy clinical process. Perhaps we will be able to determine if historical figures had ADHD by examining DNA samples from them. Thomas Edison, Leonardo di Vinci, Benjamin Franklin & Michelangelo all exhibited a number of ADHD behaviors.

In addition to these DNA studies, actual brain imaging techniques suggest the physical structure of ADHD affected brains differ from non-affected brains.[vii]

One "theory" advanced by Thom Hartmann is that ADHD behavior is the product of remnant "Hunter" DNA still in our human gene pool. This "Hunter" DNA provides humans with certain behavioral tendencies that were extremely useful during our Hunter Gatherer past, but are considered a disorder by today's industrialized society. Hartmann gives the example of the hunter who has been tracking a boar suddenly being confronted by a deer.

The hunter must choose immediately between continuing his original stalk, or change his attention to the deer he can see. He doesn't have time to consider all the possibilities or hold a planning meeting with the other members of the hunting party. He needs to choose one or the other course of action. And he needs to do it now. So is the ability to act without fully considering each possible outcome individual impulsivity, or is it a survival trait for our species?

Keep in mind Hunter Gatherer societies can still be found in isolated parts of the world today. And it was only a few thousand years ago that the majority of humans lived a Hunter

Gatherer lifestyle. Mr. Hartmann argues that the human behaviors required to support the agriculture and industrial revolutions moved these hunter behaviors from the asset side to the liability side of the human equation.

While I have seen no scholarly work legitimizing this particular theory, it has a sense of logic and appeal. ADHD is found in every society and country of the world irrespective of diet, video games, social structure, and religion. This strongly suggests the tendency toward ADHD behaviors is a human characteristic that exists in our gene pool for a reason. Just as sickle cell anemia provides those who have that condition with an increased level of protection from malaria. ADHD provides those who have the condition with a different way of seeing the world around them, one that can be an asset in athletics.

But, the true value of Thom Hartmann's premise, is it magically transposes the stigma of having a brain defect or disorder, into a positive trait. Particularly for an elementary or middle school student who has likely experienced continual criticism for his or her ADHD behaviors it is much more acceptable and affirming to consider yourself a hunter, rather than someone with a brain defect.

I would also be remiss if I did not note that a head trauma, even a relatively insignificant one without loss of consciousness, could result in ADHD type behaviors.

In my opinion, given the large and ever increasing amount of data pointing at DNA, the large majority of ADHD cases are simply the result of a roll of the genetic dice; much as red hair, left handedness, gender or sickle cell anemia are also determined at conception.

Spock's Brain & ADHD

Without understanding the basic structure and functions of the brain, it is difficult to understand how the ADHD affected brain drives ADHD behavior.[4]

100,000 years ago the typical human brain weighed about a pound. Today the typical human brain weighs about three pounds and consists of some 100 billion (1^{11}) individual brain cells or neurons.[viii] So in a relatively short evolutionary period the human brain

---

[4] Undoubtedly, many readers know more about the human brain than I. I have relied completely on the work of professionals in this area and have done my best to recognize them for this work.

experienced a threefold increase in the number of cells. This increased mass primarily occurred in the brain's cortex; the commonly recognized, corrugated outside layer of the brain. The cortex is also that area of the brain to which the behavioral issues most often associated with ADHD are traced.

Located directly behind our forehead, are the frontal lobes and our pre-frontal cortex (PFC). The primary function provided by the PFC is controlling the executive functions of our brain. These include our ability to plan and anticipate outcomes, to direct attentional resources to meet the demands of non-routine events, to provide self-monitoring and self-awareness necessary for determining the appropriateness of behavior, and for behavioral flexibility.

Additionally the PFC provides input to our time management, judgment, impulse control, multi-step sequential planning (e.g. what should I do first, second and third when tying a shoe), organization, and critical thinking. It also acts as a storage bin or bookmark for "short-term" memory. Ideally, people can keep their place on one thought while they consider another and then come back to their "bookmark". For the ADDer the "bookmark" falls out of the book much more quickly.

I like to think of the PFC as "Spock's Brain". Generally speaking, the more active this section of the brain is, the more "logical" and unflappable the individual appears. The less active this area of the brain is, the less "Spock-like" the individual behaves.

Other areas of the brain often associated with ADHD are the parietal and temporal lobes and our inner brain. The parietal lobes are the primary sensory areas (taste, touch, temperature and movement) of our brain. The temporal lobes are responsible for interpreting sounds and integrating memories and sensations such as taste, sight, sound and touch.

Finally our inner brain acts as the "gate keeper" between our spinal cord and cerebral cortex. Located in the center of our brain, the inner brain determines our emotional state, modifies our perceptions and responses and initiates movement or actions without us needing to think about them.

Neurons, Dopamine and Norepinephrine

Irrespective of the functions they perform, each part of our brain consists of individual brain cells called neurons. Functionally, a neuron is simply a binary (on/off) switch; connected to an estimated 10,000 other neurons by an intertwined network of sending (axons) and receiving (dendrites) cell components.[ix]

As you can see from the illustration, dendrites are located at one end of the neuron while the axon is a comparatively long appendage located on the other end.

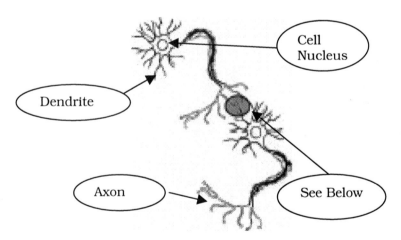

When a neuron receives a signal through it's web of dendrites, it "fires" a signal down its axon. When this signal reaches the end of the axon it triggers the release of various chemical neurotransmitters into the gap between the axon and dendrites of adjacent neurons. Ideally, this chemical release results in a signal being sent across the synaptic gap or synapse to the next neuron.

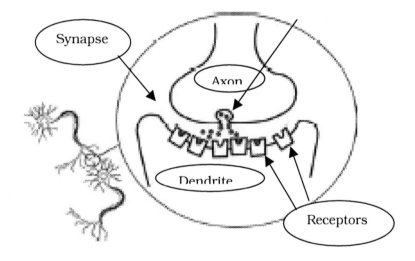

Neurotransmitters are what carry the actual signal between the cells in our body. And there are a multitude of different neurotransmitters used throughout our body. For example, the neurotransmitter acetylcholine is released where nerves meet muscles and is therefore responsible for all voluntary muscle contractions throughout our body. The neurotransmitters most often associated with ADHD are dopamine and norepinephrine.

Dopamine is strongly associated with several brain functions including planning, attention, and learning. Ideally, the neurons in the PFC have both an increased supply of dopamine and an increased number of dopamine receptors than cells in other parts of our brain. Low levels of dopamine in the PFC results in a poorly performing PFC. This in turn results in lowered levels of executive functions to the rest of the brain which influences individual behavior.

Also affecting this signaling process is the "leftover" level of a neurotransmitter that has previously been released into the synapse.

A high "leftover" level means the sending neuron has to release less of a given neurotransmitter to reach a "threshold trigger". Lower levels means more must be released to reach the "threshold trigger". If the total level (leftover + new) of the neurotransmitter is below what is needed to reach this trigger, then no signal is passed on and the information flow stops.

Medications and Scaring Deer

The most common medications used to reduce the effects of ADHD are stimulants such as methylphenidate (Ritalin) and amphetamines (Adderall or Dexedrine). Studies indicate these medications boost the levels of both serotonin and dopamine; and inhibit dopamine transporters from reducing the level of dopamine in the synapse.

One way to visualize this process is to compare it to the "shishi odoshi" or "deer scare" used by Japanese farmers to scare away deer from their crops. This is a length of bamboo with one end cut at an angle and the other end resting on a rock. A shaft is placed through the length of bamboo so the angled end is lighter than the end resting on the rock. As water fills up the angled end, it becomes heavier, the balance point shifts and bamboo tips downward. The water then runs out, the balance point shifts again and the bamboo returns to the original position. When the bamboo strikes the rock it makes a noise, scaring away deer.

The total weight of the water is what causes the center of gravity to shift, tipping the shishi odoshi. Not enough water and nothing will happen.

What if there was a leak in the bamboo? As water enters some would also leak out. The critical amount is never reached, the center of gravity never shifts and it would never tip. The bamboo would never strike the rock, scaring away the deer. The deer would eat the crop.

This is what happens in the ADDer brain. In addition to receiving less dopamine from the sending neuron, the dopamine that is in the synapse rapidly "leaks away" through the process of re-uptake.

By simultaneously increasing the level of dopamine in the neuron and inhibiting re-uptake these medications work the same as providing a greater flow of water and a temporary patch to the shishi odoshi.

"No Free Lunch"

One would think then that everyone could simply take as much of these medications as they wanted and everyone would be fine. We would all be in control of our emotions and unbothered by any distractions. But one of life's great maxims is "There is no such thing as a free lunch." Just as inadequate levels of dopamine contribute toward ADHD behaviors, excess levels of dopamine (as might occur with the abuse of some drugs such as amphetamines) in the brain have been associated with paranoia, hallucinations, delusions, agitation and mania.

While all the preceding few pages are interesting for understanding where ADHD comes from and how it affects our brain, for many of us this issue is irrelevant.

Because irrespective of it's cause ADHD is defined and determined by the behaviors of impulsivity, distractibility, inattention, lack of follow through and hyperactivity. How those around us react to these behaviors are what get, and keep, ADDers in trouble with the world.

Common Misconceptions

Some of the more common misconceptions regarding ADHD follow.

"If you only tried harder, you would..."

From the time we start school, every single ADDer hears the following liturgy from our parents, teachers, coaches, principals, and grandparents. We grew up hearing it. We still hear it.

✗ "If you only tried harder you would control your ADHD behavior."

"If you only tried harder you would wait your turn."

"If you only tried harder you wouldn't butt into conversations."

"If you only tried harder you wouldn't lose things, you would remember your bag, book, homework assignment."

"If you only tried harder you wouldn't make so many mistakes."

"If you only tried harder you would do it."

"If you only tried harder you..."

The most bewildering thing about this misconception is how many people believe ADDers fail deliberately. But if they would think for just an instant they might realize how illogical this thought is.

Despite hanging around athletes at all levels for several decades I have never met any athlete who deliberately and consciously chose to fail. I've never met the athlete who lays awake at night thinking of novel ways to lose a match, give up a touchdown, or false start during a race.

The assumption is that everyone can control his or her attentional focus and behaviors all the time. Medication, environmental controls, education and/or learning skills can modify the impact of some ADHD behaviors. But the root cause driving those behaviors, the level of neurotransmitter receptors in our brain, is not consciously controllable by us.

"ADDers don't pay attention"

The second commonly held misconception is that those suffering from ADHD can't or won't pay attention. The reality is we pay attention to everything. What we have difficulty doing is maintaining attention or focus on events, tasks or people.

Does this result from an "under performing" sensory filtering mechanism in the ADHD brain or does the sensory filtering mechanism in a non-ADHD brain "over perform"? Actually both of these views are correct, depending on what someone is doing at the moment.

What the offended is really saying is "The ADDer didn't pay attention to me when I think he or she should have paid attention to me."

"ADDers have Bad Attitudes"

Another common misconception is ADDers have a "bad attitude". Since I've never actually seen an attitude (good or bad) I always ask the speaker to define a "bad attitude". What typically happens is the speaker goes down the list of ADHD behaviors and projects his personal values onto those behaviors.

"He doesn't do what I tell him to do" or "He won't change his behavior even when he's punished" which makes him "defiant". "He doesn't pay attention when I'm talking and he interrupts me"; which makes him "disrespectful". "He's always picking fights with others" which means he is argumentative or violent.

The speaker has taken past emotional responses and transferred[5] them to the ADDer's character. If the behavior is frustrating, then the ADDer deliberately did it to frustrate me. If the behavior is rude, then it was deliberately done to insult me. If the behavior is the opposite of what I told the ADDer to do, then the ADDer is deliberately disobedient or insubordinate to me. The curious thing about this is the speaker honestly believes the ADDer acted deliberately.

---

[5] As used here, <u>transference</u> occurs when someone transfers emotions from past relationships or experiences to the present. For example, a baseball player might have been extremely angry when the right fielder on his team misplayed a fly ball in a championship game. But twenty years later as a coach he may become enraged when he notices his right fielder has started picking daisies even though (or perhaps because) no ball has been hit into right field for the last three games.

"Stimulants can't help someone control hyperactivity"

One of the great mysteries of life is how Ritalin, an amphetamine, and other psychiatric medications, result in the ADDer becoming less hyperactive, less impulsive and less distractible. Intuitively it should make ADDers more hyperactive.

In a non-medicated or non-hyperfocus[6] state ADDers scan everything. Sensory input to an ADDer works like a motion alarm where any movement automatically (subconsciously) moves to the top of the list for our attention or consideration.

Stimulant medications, such as Ritalin or Adderall, change or slow the prioritizing process from automatic to semi-automatic. So instead of being at the mercy of the process, the ADDer can finish one task before moving onto another.

---

[6] Hyper-focus occurs when an ADDer becomes totally focused with responding to a set of visually stimulating tasks, such as a video or computer game. As someone once noted, "There is no ADHD in front of a good video game."

Keep in mind that ADHD is a condition of awareness of what is going on around you. When I was diagnosed and began taking medication I was stunned at how easy it was to disregard external stimuli and stay on task long enough to finish things.

Often I didn't even notice the external stimuli that had **shrieked** at me before. Without those interruptions, I had a better chance of finishing things when they were supposed to be finished. But with those distractions I seemed to spend most of my time trying to get back to what I was doing before I was interrupted by the distraction.

Writing a book in the past was an impossible task for me. Now, instead of a continuous search for which page I was on, writing a book is nothing but a matter of time and effort.

"People outgrow ADHD as they get older"

While once it was thought to be a childhood condition, ADHD is generally now accepted to be a lifetime human condition. In the past, it seemed to disappear at adulthood. I suspect what really occurred is that those suffering the condition simply found jobs and careers that suited their condition. Often such jobs were physically demanding, outdoor work. But, in the early 21st century (with an ever increasingly technologically based economy) many of these jobs and careers have been eliminated or transferred from our society.

Another career previously open to ADDers was the military. Many ADDers actually excelled in military service because of the structure it imposes. Many of the choices that exist outside the military (what clothes to wear, when to leave for work, what to eat, etc.) simply don't exist inside the military. Making the wrong choice among a multitude of options can lead to problems for the ADDer. In a tightly controlled environment, there is less chance to make the wrong choice. Indeed, there may not be any choice to make.

Unfortunately ADDers are often discouraged from joining the service in large part because in peacetime the military does not permit the use of common ADHD medications, even under a prescription. This is, in my opinion, somewhat shortsighted because during actual combat operations the military often issue service members "go pills" (reportedly simple amphetamines).

ADDers also develop coping mechanisms for their condition. Some of these mechanisms are more successful than others; and some cases of ADHD are simply more severe than others. But people generally do not outgrow it.

"ADDers won't do as they're told"

Actually, most ADDers do as they are told, it is just they may not do exactly as they are told. When we are told something we likely hear it differently than how the speaker intended. Remember one of the identifying symptoms is an inability to process verbal instructions into action.

One of the curious things about being an ADDer is the ability to come up with new solutions to old problems. Some of the most creative people in our time display ADDer behaviors. If you can't stay on task for extended periods of time, how can you come up with new solutions to old problems? Because ADDers spend so much time in a scanning mode.... looking for something new or stimulating...we are used to coming back to problems that we were distracted from. When we come back to the original problem it often appears differently than when we got distracted. So we perceive things differently and may come to different solutions.

"Isn't this just the newest media disease?"

ADHD was first described in a scientific journal in 1902 as "Still's disease". There have also been numerous observations of people in almost all societies who exhibit ADHD behavior. The condition has long been recognized and written about in a variety of cultures, though not necessarily as ADHD. Many have thought that MacBeth exhibited classic ADHD behaviors. Some traditional cultures such as India, Japan, and native hunting societies in North America all value the behaviors. Others, typically more industrialized western cultures, feel the behaviors are a disorder.

"Isn't this just a way to sell drugs to kids?"

This is really just a different spin on the previous question. As stated early over 6 million K-12 students in our country receive medication in order to function in our schools. But given crowded classrooms and a decreasing emphasis on physical activity, what would happen without medication? If teachers have difficulty teaching over thirty students in a room with ADHD medication, how much more difficult would a teacher have without these medications? Always remember, only a medical doctor, can prescribe these medications.

"Is there a cure for ADHD?"

No more than a cure exists for diabetes, color blindness or sickle cell anemia. ADHD is defined to the world as a cluster of human behaviors. And while education, behavior modification, and medication may lessen the impact of these behaviors in some environments, the primary driver is the level of neurotransmitters received across the synaptic gap between brain cells. There is no "cure".

"Then how can an ADDer athlete be successful?"

ADHD is a lifelong condition driven primarily by the levels of certain neurotransmitters in specific parts of the brain. These levels significantly affect how ADDers perceive and respond to their immediate environment. Labeling these perceptions and responses as good or bad misses the essential point. ADHD exists and isn't going to magically "go away". Therefore, the best way for an ADHD affected athlete to become "successful" is to learn how to take advantage of the condition.

Anyone, ADDer or not, is more likely be successful by learning to use the gifts they do have rather than trying to develop gifts they don't have. For example, no matter how hard he worked at it, Michael Jordan was an average, minor league baseball player. He simply did not have the physical gifts to play MLB. But what were liabilities in the batters box turned into priceless assets on a basketball court.

Because ADHD isn't going to "go away", the primary objective for the parent or coach of an ADDer must be to encourage and support the athlete in finding and developing ways to take advantage of what ADHD gives to the athlete, rather than telling the athlete to stop being ADHD.

How ADHD Affects People

Hitting .400

There is a story that a sportswriter once asked Ted Williams (major league baseball's last .400 hitter) what was his secret for hitting a baseball. Ted responded that he could tell if a pitch was a curve, changeup or fastball within a few feet of the ball leaving the pitcher's hand by simply watching the rotation of the red stitching on the seams of the baseball. Ted then asked the reporter why he was asking a question with such an obvious answer. What Ted Williams didn't fully understand until later in his life was his "normal vision" was for the rest of the world supernormal.

But Ted Williams' visual ability significantly shaped his perception of other players' effort and character. Since Ted's only experience was seeing the world through his remarkable eyes, he logically assumed everyone else did too. If other players didn't hit as well as he did, it was because they either chose not to or they simply didn't work as hard at hitting as he did. They were just plain lazy.

This same logical process lays the foundation for most of the interpersonal and social problems experienced by the ADHD affected. This "logic" leads people to assume everyone perceives and processes information the same way that "I" do. And, since "I" can control my behaviors by choice, so can other people. "If you really wanted to you would do it. But you're just lazy and looking for an excuse for your behavior." And given there are no visible signs of the condition, such as accompany a physical birth defect, it is completely understandable to conclude ADHD isn't a real condition, that the person is just using it as an excuse for their behavior. After all, everyone exhibits ADHD behaviors at times.

But while "normal" people effectively control their behaviors, ADDers may require medication, accommodations and/or significant job modifications. And incidentally, this is exactly what people who have poor eyesight or diabetes do. They get glasses/contacts or they take insulin that allows them to function "normally".

Who does ADHD affect? ✳

The following statement might be difficult for the reader to understand. But it is a critical concept for understanding the affect of ADHD on those who have the condition.

✳People with ADHD are unaffected by the condition directly. It only affects us indirectly through other people's actions.

How can this be?

Just as someone who is colorblind is unaware of his or her condition until they are diagnosed, it is possible for ADDers to be unaware of having ADHD until being diagnosed. And this diagnosis might not occur until the person is well into adulthood; it may not ever occur.

The people who are most affected by ADHD don't actually have the condition, but interact with ADDers. These people include teachers, family members, friends, teammates and coworkers. The affect occurs when assignments are turned in late, not at all or not even started. Completed work is often ✳ marginally acceptable, disorganized, lacks attention to detail and with obvious mistakes throughout. Seemingly simple instructions are not followed.   Meetings and deadlines are forgotten.

ADDers are aware that people around us routinely express ever-increasing levels of disappointment, frustration, anger, indifference and eventual rejection of us for what we did, didn't or forgot to do. ADHD only affects ADDers through the "punishment" of this response cycle.

What maintains this cycle is the persistent belief, sometimes even amongst our families that ADHD is either a "convenient excuse for laziness" or that ADDers really can overcome the condition if we really wanted to.

"You are what you do."

In addition to the personal criticism from the individuals around us regarding "what" we did, didn't or forgot to do, is an underlying societal condemnation of the behaviors.

One of America's social values is "You are what you do"; that each one of us fully controls our behaviors and becomes "successful" through self-discipline, self-determination, attention to detail and hard work.

This socialization starts early with childhood stories such as "The Ant and the Grasshopper" or "The Tortoise and the Hare." The fundamental message from both of these stories is that the "good person" stays focused on the same job day after day, not noticing or being pulled away from the task at hand. The "bad person" is the one who doesn't pay attention, doesn't finish what he or she starts, and is invariably overtaken in the end by the "good person".

Unmentioned in these stories is that the rabbit will likely be eaten by predators unless he remains fully aware of everything going on around him. Or that the tortoise's response to every danger is to pull his head and feet into a shell and pretend the danger isn't there.

Nor is it mentioned that the only purpose served by a worker ant is to gather food for higher-ranking ants in the nest. These "higher-ranking" ants, and not the worker ants, are the ones living in the best part of the nest and breeding with the queen.[7]

---

[7] If you never thought of these points before, you now have some idea of how easy it is for the ADDer to get into trouble with bureaucratic authority, particularly when observations such as these are impulsively blurted out in a school classroom to a teacher who doesn't expect or like to be challenged.

So when the defining behaviors of ADHD inevitably collide with these social values (most often triggered by repeatedly disappointing an employer, teacher, school administrator, parent or athletic coach) the ADHD affected individual is perceived as having flawed values and character.

Subsequently ADDers are viewed as rude, insensitive, selfish, aggressive, defiant, insubordinate, disrespectful, deceitful, untrustworthy, apathetic, and lazy.

By recognizing this simple process, the reader can begin to appreciate why ADDers are so often considered to be generally "bad people".

ADDers become ostracized by the very society to which we belong. And this rejection in turn contributes to any number of social problems for ADDers including a sense of rejection by society, emotional isolation, depression, distrust, anxiety, beliefs of inferiority, sense of failure, and often an underlying anger or even rage.

It is essential to understand that these are not deliberate behaviors on the part of the ADHD affected athlete and there is no reason to respond as if they were. These behaviors aren't something we can willfully turn on or off, anymore than the reader can willfully stop seeing in color.

Biggest Challenge Faced by ADHD Athletes

What is the biggest challenge facing the ADHD affected athlete? Is it inattention, impulsiveness, lack of organization, or hyperactivity?

The biggest problem is the coach, who becomes so concerned with controlling what the athlete does on the field or court, that they forget every sport is about the athlete reaching his or her potential. Any mistake is seemingly taken as a deliberate challenge to the coach's authority. But sports are not about the coach. They are about the athlete.

Unfortunately we have all seen the stereotypical basketball coach's behavior after one of his players commits a particularly egregious error. The coach invariably leaps to his feet waving his arms around; possibly talks to his assistant, maybe cursing, maybe appealing for divine intervention by outstretching his hands and looking up to heaven, and often calling a time out.

The next step is to substitute in "the new player". When the offending player comes out, the coach typically asks several nonsensical rhetorical questions of the offending player "What were you thinking?" "How could you let that player do that to you?"

The coach then banishes the player to exile at the far end of the bench with a nod of their head or gesture from their hand. Alternatively the coach might simply ignore the player, as he or she walks toward basketball's St. Helena.

Such public actions by the coach would lead one to assume the athlete deliberately chose to make an error, as if engaged in some weird Machiavellian scheme to embarrass the coach or sabotage the team. Maybe the athlete laid awake the night before scheming on how to publicly screw up so the coach would become angry. Perhaps even downloading new ways to fail at www.how2screwup.com. After such an outburst, the player is embarrassed, his or her teammates are embarrassed, and the fans are embarrassed.

Life can be tough without ADHD. It's tougher with ADHD. It's tougher still with ADHD and a coach who believes you deliberately made a mistake to publicly embarrass or defy him or her. And there are many ways for an athlete to respond to this coaching behavior. Unfortunately one common response is to x avoid the situation all together by retiring.

This is okay when an athlete is thirty. But when the athlete is fourteen with ADHD it is a theft of opportunity and experience for the athlete.

This is another of society's crimes against the ADHD affected athlete, the crime of conforming or rejection. It is also one of society's crimes against itself. Because one place an ADDer can be him or her self, where his or her condition can be unleashed in a positive manner is in athletics. If you, as a coach, sincerely want the ADHD affected athlete to succeed, then help them embrace their gifts rather than reject them.

For coaches who are willing to look, ADHD offers athletes remarkable gifts, particularly in sports with high levels of chaos, which is the fundamental state of existence for most ADDers. Coaches who are unable to recognize and embrace these gifts will never be able to bring out the potential in ADHD affected athletes.

Advantages of ADHD

Is ADHD always a liability, particularly to athletes? In the right circumstances ADHD may provide unexpected advantages to athletes.

Much as a blind person gains a heightened sense of smell and hearing, ADDers can develop a heightened awareness of their immediate environment. This awareness offers athletes the potential for a more adaptive response to certain sports than the non-ADHD affected possess.

If their coach encourages them, ADHD affected athletes may develop an ability to look at their sport with a different perspective, seeing different ways to play the game and the confidence to try it in competitive situations.

Snipe

When I was in high school I watched a wrestler work out in the Multnomah Athletic Club in Portland, Oregon. Where every other wrestler I had seen gave no advantage to their opponent;

this wrestler's basic stance was to put one of his legs directly in front of his opponent and literally taunt his opponent to take it.

Curious, I asked him why he wrestled that way. At the time I thought his reply indicated his head had been bounced off the floor too many times. Today I see an incredible insight into his sport and the psychology of his opponents. He recognized wrestlers were coached to avoid risk, and not give any opportunity to their opponent. In such situations, neither wrestler had an obvious opportunity. And both had to defend against a variety of possible attacks. But his approach forced his opponent to one offensive option; the single leg takedown.

So instead of having to defend against any number of possible attacks he only had to defend against that one technique. And defending against one technique was much more efficient. And his opponent began thinking what to do instead of just wrestling.

He also practiced for hours wrestling from unique situations. He would then lead or force his opponent into those situations during matches. Situations that he was comfortable and relaxed with, but where his opponent was tentative and cautious.

Subsequently he was always more confident and relaxed than his opponent. His situational awareness of where he and his opponent were always located on the mat was (for lack of a better term) eerie, almost creepy.

I have a photo of his last tournament where he had mastered this technique to the point where he was standing on one leg and actually pushing his opponent off the mat by putting his other foot onto his opponent's chest. The wrestler's name was Rick Sanders and at the time I met him he had won a pair of NCAA championships at Portland State University, a silver medal at the Mexico City Olympics, and a world championship in Argentina. The picture I have was from the Munich Olympics where he won a second silver medal. Several people who knew him well have assured me Rick was the most ADHD affected athlete they had ever met or dealt with.

Impulsivity-Fearlessness

While many consider impulsivity to be a negative trait, in the right situation it is a positive trait. Someone who always looks before they leap, or considers all the possible actions before implementing the best one, may seldom make a mistake or fail. But it is unlikely they will be successful in those athletic contests that reward the competitor who initiates the action, even if it isn't the "best choice". Speed of response is the great equalizer. A closely related trait to impulsivity is a general sense of fearlessness in a time of crisis or stimulation. ADDers simply aren't overly concerned with long-term possibilities, or consequences of their actions. Some ADDers may actually seek out such stimulation and exciting situations.

ADDers are 'hard wired' to instantaneously process information and take a course of action. ADDers do not agonize over the process, hold a meeting to discuss all the alternatives, and select the one with the best cost/reward ratio. Generally speaking, ADDers do not feel guilty for being themselves, nor do they understand everyone else's aversion to "just doing it".

Situational Awareness

Another trait ADDers seem to share is situational awareness or vision. "Coach he was open. He just didn't know it" is a classic ADDer explanation. Many people believe

ADDers aren't paying attention to what goes on around them. But the reality is quite different. The reality is we are aware of almost everything going on around us.

I freely admit I do not know what it is like not to have ADHD. After all I was born with it. But I believe it is worth sharing the lack of awareness I experience when I am on medication compared to when I am not. When I take a walk in my neighborhood med free I subconsciously scan everything in sight from the front door of one house to the front door of the house across the street. The street itself is just empty space between lawns. I note different species of birch trees, mushrooms growing in a lawn, different shades of green paint on the same house where someone didn't properly mix the paint together before applying it. I wonder if that will have an impact on the life of the siding beneath the paint. I hear cats fighting, a car three blocks away going too fast. I smell both the first fireplace fire of the season and the last barbeque. In short, I am aware of what is going on around me.

Yet when I take that same walk when I am on medication I notice the sidewalk in front of me. My awareness ends at the curb and the edge of the lawn. It is almost as though a bell jar has been placed around me, limiting my awareness to a few feet on either side. I have to consciously look, listen, and smell the environment around me, rather than being part of it.

Scanning

Perhaps the easiest way to understand how ADDers receive external information is to compare our attention span to an emergency radio scanner. Such scanners automatically cycle through the various frequencies, playing each one for a few seconds, and then moving to the next. This is remarkably similar to the way ADDers receive information. Everything around us is unconsciously scanned for interest or importance. If nothing is of interest we move on to the next "channel". So not only does an ADDer hear the news, weather reports, and traffic alerts; we also tune in briefly to the police dispatcher and ambulances. But while this scanning goes on, we are attempting to function in the society around us. Unfortunately all too often teachers, parents, coaches and bosses perceive this scanning as not paying attention.

Assume a football coach is lecturing his team on a particular point when he notices one of his players isn't "paying attention." The coach assumes the player is daydreaming. The reality is the ADDer is simply scanning his environment and notices a number of things in just 15 seconds. He noticed a teammate scratching his ear, a car going by on the road (right rear tire is low), the janitor is sweeping down the court (broom handle is cracked and someone put tape on it, blue masking tape), a girl with red tights running on the track, the seagull flying behind her, there must be a storm blowing in, he wonders how she gets the tights on, he checks in to see if the coach has gotten to a point, nope still talking about when he was playing, he wonders if the coach knows his shoe laces don't match, who is the girl with the red tights running on the track, etc., etc., etc.

ADDers go through each day continuously scanning everything around us. But before we get into the details of any particular item, we likely notice something else. If someone is speaking (particularly in an environment with a lot of things going on such as a practice field) and they don't get to the point quickly, we likely are paying attention to something else.

Scanning works well for noting the unmarked forward at the far post, that a linebacker has his feet mixed up and can be beaten to the outside, or that the defenders on the hockey team you are playing missed their last line change and are spent physically.

It is probably less adaptable for gymnastics, diving, swimming (but great for water polo) or distance running (steeple chase and cross country excepted).

The Empty Mind and "The Zone"

"You are the spectator by the great stream. A wave rises, it is noticed. Your opponent moves, no mind follows. The hundred things--the dark winged messengers of your psyche entice you--pulses of light transport you--you do not resist because nothing is in the way. Simply you are here, observing mind and things are as they are."[x]

Mushin is a Japanese Martial arts term that doesn't translate well into English. Literally it means "Empty mind" or "No mind". But the connotations attached to it suggest a more accurate translation is "The Emptied or Ready Mind."

Kendo, the martial art of Japanese fencing, strongly encourages developing this state of awareness where the Kendoist has emptied every conscious thought, intent and emotion from his or her mind, opening it completely to the match or training. Both the match and training go on, but Mushin lets one be aware of doing it, instead of telling themselves to do it. In Western Culture this state of mine is referred to as being in "the Zone".

At one time or another most athletes have entered "the Zone". When athletes are in "the Zone" the basketball rim looks 4 feet across and they wait for a 95 MPH fastball to get to the plate. The Zone is where your body does it, without being consciously told to do anything.

My youngest son refers to "the Zone" as a place where everyone and everything slows down, where in full stride he can "one touch" a bouncing soccer ball 35 yards across the field to a teammate's shooting foot, while simultaneously stepping over a defender's slide tackle at his knee.

When I served as a U.S. Naval officer one of my jobs required me to routinely qualify at the pistol range on North Island, across the bay from San Diego. Several times I remember reaching a point of non-awareness where the target's bulls eye seemed to balance on the front sight. My finger would squeeze the trigger between heartbeats that I could see on that front sight.

Such descriptions create a shared vision of what this altered state of awareness is and is not.

Every time I've experienced, read about or listened to an athlete talking about being in "the Zone" the words control, planning and thought are never mentioned.

What athletes do speak about is experiencing a sense of timelessness, of calm certainty, without any fear of making a mistake. The athlete's perception of time changes, narrowing to the knife-edge of now, without a past or future. In the zone, the athlete's body acts without control, planning or instruction from the brain. It is as though the athlete's consciousness is simply along for the ride.

But control, planning and conscious intent are executive functions of the brain, which reside in the brain's PFC region. Given the lack of "executive controls" associated with ADHD, it is reasonable to conclude the ADHD athlete operates closer to this altered state of consciousness than the non-ADDer does. The non-ADHD athlete must get his or her conscious mind out of the way before they can enter "the Zone". Often for the ADDer, it is already out of the way.

But while the cost of admittance into "the Zone" might be discounted by the ADHD affected athlete's sense of awareness, eviction from the zone is just a distracted thought away.

Attentional Focus Styles

Dr. Robert Nideffer[xi] has developed a useful model to examine the effect of concentration styles on sports. A pair of bisected vertical and horizontal lines represents this model. The vertical axis represents narrow to broad concentration. The horizontal axis represents depth of concentration, external to internal.

This diagram creates four quadrants. The upper right quadrant represents Broad/Internal focus of concentration. This would be used to kick, hit or catch a ball in sport.

The lower right quadrant represents Narrow/Internal focus of concentration such as a diver or high jumper would use in focusing very narrowly on a specific act or routine and visually rehearsing that routine mentally before performing it.

The lower left quadrant represents Narrow/External focus of concentration such as a coach would use in analyzing who to play or what changes to make as the game occurs.

The upper left quadrant represents Broad/External focus of concentration where the athlete must be simultaneously aware of and react to what is occurring throughout the field of play. This is the quadrant where the ADHD affected athlete would be most comfortable.

It is important to recognize that while everyone shifts in and out of each one of these quadrants during the course of a competition, each one of us is most comfortable operating in one of these styles. It is also important to recognize that each sport rewards the different concentration style to a greater or lesser degree.

If one places individual and team sports on this model, based on the primary concentration style required to perform the skill sets of that sport, an interesting pattern emerges.

For example, low chaos sports such as diving, high jumping, figure skating, and gymnastics events occur in the lower, right quadrant. These are Narrow/Internal focus events.

Competitors have no direct effect on one another's success in such sports. Indeed competitors are prohibited from preventing one another from succeeding. A high jumper doesn't have to worry about being tackled by a competitor during his approach to the bar. A figure skater doesn't have to worry about a competitor "hip-checking" her into the boards as she sets up for a jump. Time, distance and the "style" score of judges determine who wins or loses in such activities.

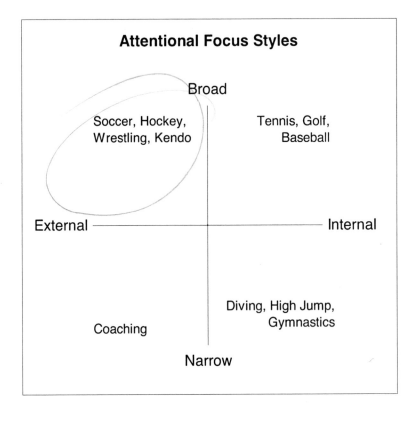

Attentional Focus Styles

Broad

Soccer, Hockey,
Wrestling, Kendo

Tennis, Golf,
Baseball

External ——————————————— Internal

Coaching

Diving, High Jump,
Gymnastics

Narrow

But in the upper left quadrant are sports with high chaos levels, where head to head competitors directly affect the outcome. Time, distance, and judge's "style points" have no impact on the outcome of a match between two heavyweight boxers or an ice hockey game (which some might consider the same sport).

The type of coaching given to a gymnast between vaults is likely much different than that given to a hockey player between shifts. Coaches who are technique oriented (Lower/Right quadrant) or who are inclined to directly control the contest need to be aware of their tendencies when communicating with ADHD affected athletes (Upper/Left quadrant). Also keep in mind that miscommunications can be magnified when one athlete is ADHD affected and the coach and another is not.

Keys to Coaching ADHD Affected Athletes

The following from an ADHD diagnosed fencer covers key elements in coaching ADHD affected athletes.

"I have thought about why I like the structure of my coaches' lesson and concluded that they are most like doing yoga; it is mindful exercise. The repetition becomes almost trance like. The mind is engaged in feeling and controlling the muscles and breathing. I am never bored.

Also, my coach carries a tremendous personal intensity and he rarely speaks during the session. All of his students become riveted to his physical movements. He'll change his preparations suddenly without notice, yet he gives the student time to catch up until they work as one unit.

Personally, I seem to have better than usual retention for what he teaches me. Intellectually, he explores other areas, portions of time within or around an action, in a seemingly logical manner, without discussion or explanation, yet it is so obvious that this is the meat of the lesson. Two activities are happening at one time.

Through the physical repetition, I build muscle memory around a skill set and I become more confident to use those skills in a bout situation. The more comfortable I feel about my physical base of technical training, the better I feel about competing. I respond more favorably to unexpected situations. It all fits together so neatly."

Graciously reprinted with permission of the United States Fencing Association.

The fundamental challenge facing the coach of an ADHD affected athlete is helping the athlete harness their sense of awareness and it's accompanying distractibility.

The levels of certain neurotransmitters cause the brains of ADHD affected people to work differently than the brains of non-ADHD affected work. This difference results in shorter attention span, easy distractibility, impulsivity, reactivity and difficulty in moderating physical activity. Whether the root cause of this condition is genetic, environmental, diet or the result of a head trauma is irrelevant to the coach's challenge and the athlete's success.

The reality is these differences exist. And because of this reality, a coach may need to change the manner in which information is presented to the athlete.

Communicating with the ADHD Athlete

Fundamentally, coaching is an exercise in communicating your experiences and knowledge to provide athletes with new skills and techniques. But ADHD athletes differ from non-ADHD athletes not only in how our brains are structured, how we process information, and our defining behaviors, but also in how we communicate and learn. Failure to recognize and adapt to this reality will result in you not being able to communicate your experiences and knowledge. And you will fail as a coach.

What happens if you ask a question in English to someone who only speaks Norwegian? Nothing happens because the Norwegian doesn't understand what you are saying. And asking the same question only louder doesn't change that situation.

Reportedly American born soccer players playing professionally in Germany are given an interpreter for a period of time and force-fed the language, culture and style of play.

In addition to visually drawing plays, and physically walking Yao Ming to where he was supposed to be on the court, the Houston Rockets hired a full time translator for him. Simply put, would Yao Ming be as effective today had his coaches at Houston not gone the extra mile to communicate with him early on?

This is not to say every ADDer has the talent to be Yao Ming or a professional soccer player. Nor is it suggesting Yao Ming or American soccer players in Europe are or aren't ADHD affected. The fastest way to communicate with someone is to find a common "language" for both coach and athlete.

Does it make more sense for a coach to learn how to communicate with an ADHD affected athlete or for the athlete to learn to communicate with the coach? Given the difficulty most ADDers have in our society, I suggest faster results would occur with the coach rather than the ADDer taking the lead.

What are the keys for communication with ADHD affected athletes?

Visual processor

Most ADDers react strongly to visual events and cues. Just a few of these include "post-it" reminders, visible schedules, drawings on clipboards, or videotapes. And the term "out of sight, out of mind" was almost certainly written by an ADDer. And if something is put away in a drawer, it is being "hidden" from us.

One of the things I learned from the Wild Bunch was to visually simplify communications. The team ended up with just two plays, "pick & roll" or "give & go". Whoever had the ball either held up a fist, "pick & roll" or an open palm, "give & go". They ran those two plays in some odd places, but they were all on the same page and it worked for them. Show pictures, use a chalkboard, or draw plays in the dirt.

One of the enduring images of playing football in the streets is the play drawn in the dirt or gravel. "I'm the bottle cap, I'll throw it to you (the cigarette filter) and you pitch it back to Tim (a colored rock)." Surprisingly this can be a better way to convey something to ADHD affected athletes than talking to them.

Another time honored tradition in sports is "the sign" in baseball. ADHD affected athletes easily understand all of these examples of visual communication.

Eye Contact

Wait until you have eye contact before you start speaking, show a technique or make a point. Be systematic when speaking to a team. Shift eye contact with a different player every five to eight seconds. The team will learn to attend to what you are saying. Keep it short and get to the point, quickly.

Learning By Doing, Not Watching

ADDers learn best by doing. Watching others do something or hearing a lecture doesn't get it done. We are experiential learners, we learn by trial and error.

Keep Your Messages Short & Simple

After you gain eye contact, positively KISS (Keep It Simple Stupid) the athlete. Which is easier to understand? "Mike, don't let their post take up inside position on your weak side." or "Mike, don't let him put one foot in the paint." Remember one of the definitive issues with ADDers is difficulty in understanding the intent of sequential verbal instructions. So giving the ADHD athlete a lengthy verbal instruction with multiple steps is a recipe for failure. The athlete will either forget the first part of the message, or simply not process the information into a coherent course of action.

Make Positive Statements ✗

One of the best coaches I know, Mr. Robbie Baarts, once showed what a positive statement could do. During a game at Sunset High School in Beaverton, Oregon a player missed a "tap in" goal on an open far post. (The keeper and last defender had gotten tangled up outside the near post). In an effort to "make a statement" the player "firmly struck" the ball as it lay about fifteen feet from the open goal. It rocketed over the cross bar, over the fence, over a narrow parking lot, over the power lines, landing on a car across the street some fifty yards away; promptly setting off the car's alarm.

Many coaches would immediately start berating the player for such a blunder. And, when Coach Baarts signaled the player over to the bench, everyone in the stands assumed he was going to do exactly that and possibly pull the player from the game. But when the player got to the sideline, the coach put his hands on the player's shoulders, looked him in the eye and spoke a few words.

They both started laughing.

Then the coach signaled the player to go back out onto the field. When asked later on what had been said the player responded, "Coach said the shot was perfect, but that I should use it from just a little further out; maybe midfield. Then he told me to go shoot another one."

Tell ADHD Affected Athletes to Succeed

One thing coaches continually do with ADHD athletes is tell them what not to do; "Don't screw up", or "Don't drop the ball." The underlying assumption is that by emphasizing what the athlete shouldn't do, the athlete will remember what to do. But considering many ADHD affected athletes often have a data bank full of criticism and low self-esteem, throwing another negative expectation at the athlete simply continues the cycle. Is any purpose served by throwing another negative expectation at the athlete?

Example: In a close basketball game your star guard has just fouled out. The only player left on the bench is an ADDer who has played little during the season. The player's opponent is a good player who loves to drive to the basket, but has a marginal jump shot. What should you tell your player to do? Do you say, "This is your big chance, so don't screw it up. Do not let that guy drive past you to the hoop! If he does, you'll be right back here on the bench." And as he walks onto the court you shout just loud enough for others to hear "Don't space out on me out there, we need you to stay focused."

Or do you look him straight in the eye and say "Just play defense like you've been doing all week in practice. Move your feet, keep him in front of you and let him take the jumper. Let the ref make the call."

In the first example the ADHD athlete hears that you think he will "let" his opponent score, or he will choose to lose focus and screw up that way. In any event you, his coach, expect him to fail.

In the second example, the coach gave him some very clear instructions of what to do based on what he had been doing in practice. The coach also encouraged the player to do something. And at the end he took any fear of failure away by making the referee responsible for the call.

Which coach will get the better performance from the same player?

Verify What You Said

ADDers are great at appearing to pay rapt attention to what coaches, teachers and parents are saying. It is an acquired skill. So you may think what you are saying has "sunk in". Maybe it has, and maybe it hasn't. The only way you will know before the game is to ask. If you don't verify what you said, you have no idea if they understood it or not.

Ask the athletes to repeat back what they heard you say. Ask them what it means. The question to ask is not "What did I say?" The question to ask is "What did you hear me say?" And there is a difference between those two questions. What you said is irrelevant. What the athlete heard you say is what he or she will do.

Give Unqualified Praise

Hand out buckets of unqualified praise as if your boat is sinking into shark-infested water. Start today. Do it tomorrow. Keep doing it. Look for actions and efforts to praise. Do it as often as you can. Give out praise for effort and for "on task behavior". And best results come from small, frequent praise over the course of training or competition.

"Tim, great effort forcing him to his left. Well done!" "Keep up the hard work and effort."

Remember the ADHD affected athlete has spent much of his or her life being criticized for simply being him or herself. Giving legitimate praise to an ADDer is putting fuel into a tank that has probably been running on fumes for some time. Fill it up and you will get maximum effort in return.

Qualifying Praise

One of the great thefts performed by coaches on all athletes, but on ADDers in particular, is giving praise with one breath and then taking it away with the next, by adding a qualifier. The assumption seems to be the qualifier "motivates" the athlete. But the ADDer likely doesn't hear the praise for what was accomplished; only the criticism of what wasn't accomplished. Qualifiers steal self-esteem and any sense of accomplishment from the ADDer, leaving self-doubt and a sense of failure in their place.

A 200-meter sprinter finishes second in a race and runs a personal record, 2/10th of a second off the club record. After the race the coach says the following. "Sue, you ran a great race and got a PR (personal record)!" And then the qualifier "I know you can beat that gal next time. If you run the turn just a little harder, you can break the club record too." What the coach thinks he is doing is congratulating the runner, showing confidence in her abilities and motivating her for the next race. But the ADHD runner likely hears the following. "Sue, you didn't win and I think you should have because I know you can beat that gal. And if you weren't so lazy on the turn you would have set a club record."

Don't mix motivation and showing confidence in with praise. For ADDers in particular they are separate issues. "Sue, you ran a great race and got a PR. Well done!" And then shut up! Save the motivation and improvement for the next training session, which is when people work on getting better, not during the celebration.

One soccer player once shared with me the biggest reason he had "retired" at age 16 was because no matter what he accomplished (including Olympic Development Program) it was never enough. There was always a criticism of what he hadn't done. If he scored two goals, he was reminded of the missed shot. If he got three assists, he was interrogated about why he didn't take the open shot. When he quit the sport he told both his coach and parents, "If I scored three goals in the final of the World Cup, and my team lost you would say "Too bad, if you had worked a little harder you might have won." The real shame in this incident was the player was absolutely correct in his view.

The Rhetorical Question

The greatest threat to athletic success is a drumbeat of constant criticism in the form of the reinforcement of failing to meet expectations, of simply not being good enough. This isn't constructive or honest criticism. Rather it is an abuse of power by the coach asking a "Rhetorical Question."

"What were you thinking?"

"How can you not get this done, it's so simple?"

"How can you let him beat you?"

ADHD athletes have likely lived with this type of criticism more than any other group of athletes. It has been asked of us by parents and teachers, likely for as far back as we can recall. Missed assignments, silly mistakes, lost schoolwork, accusations of "day dreaming", not applying ourselves, and the unspoken or spoken accusation of just being lazy.

I once overheard a soccer coach criticize a goalkeeper at the first practice following a 1-1 tie. The other team had scored in the last few minutes of the game when they pushed everyone forward in an effort to score the equalizer.

After haranguing the effort of the entire team, he turned to the keeper and (completely ignoring the two point blank shots the keeper had stopped in the instant before the goal), asked, "How could you let that last shot in? Can any of you tell me how that could happen?"

Without hesitation one of that team's ADHD players, who I knew from another sport, impulsively replied (is there any other way?) "Poor coaching?"

I thought it was the perfect answer for what the coach was doing at that moment.

Don't ask rhetorical questions unless you want a rhetorical answer. And if you get a rhetorical answer, have the grace to smile and realize you had it coming.

Shouting Instructions & Corrections

Athletes know when they've made a mistake in competition. Usually their opponent has pointed it out to them before the coach has a chance to say a word. So shouting instructions or corrections on technique at an athlete from across the field, mat or court to point out a mistake the ADDer is already aware of serves little purpose but to "rub salt into the wound".

One question each coach asks is what to say while a competition is going on. By all means have a passion for the sport and your athletes, encourage them, make adjustments as the contest unfolds. For example, the defensive back coach may well tell a cornerback to back off the line of scrimmage as the game winds down, not wanting to give up a long pass. But shouting out individual instructions, to ADHD affected athletes in particular, may do more harm than good. I suggest it is more productive to talk with the athlete when they are not in the contest rather than "micro-managing" the athlete during the contest.

I once observed Maurice Cheeks, coach of the Portland Trailblazers, pull a player from the game just seconds after he put him into the game. The player, visibly upset with being pulled so quickly from the game, sat in the chair next to coach Cheeks. The coach turned his chair to face the player, spoke briefly, and quickly drew something on a clipboard, which he showed to the player. The player nodded his head and was sent right back into the game. In the next few minutes the player made a number of plays including a key steal, blocked a shot and several rebounds.

If the coach's objective is to encourage the athlete to perform as they have been coached to perform during training, giving the athlete specific instructions in the game is counter productive. Because the athlete is being forced to think more, rather than less. And thinking keeps the brain in the way of athletic performance.

"Walk your talk"

ADDers notice things about their coaches. They particularly notice what coaches say versus what they do. So if you make a rule or say you are going to do something you had better follow through on it. I learned this with the Wild Bunch when I started to disregard one of my own rules; if you missed or were late for practice you didn't start the next game.

Demonstrate self-control and your athletes will learn self-control. Demonstrate emotional explosiveness and that is what your athletes will demonstrate. If you say not to be disrespectful to referees, it obligates you to control your emotions when talking to a referee. If you get into the referee's face and yell at them, then your credibility to correct ADDers for doing the same thing is zip. Which brings us to discipline.

Discipline

The classical definition of discipline is helping someone learn or helping him or her down that path. It is not, as modern society has made it, doing what you are told without question. For the coach of ADHD affected athletes, discipline is providing an environment or structure in which the athlete can become successful.

Fundamental to the ADDer trial and error learning style is experiencing consequences for behavioral choices. Some of these consequences are natural. A competitor usually administers the natural consequence of an athlete not mastering fundamental techniques. The natural consequence of a boxer dropping his right hand up is an opponent's left hook to the ear. The natural consequence of a basketball player not moving his feet on defense is an opponent going by them.

The natural consequence of missing practice or a team meeting is administered as part of the progressive discipline that every good coach has.

Remember; "ADHD is a condition, not an excuse."

Build Relationships with Athletes

Try to spend individual time each practice with the athlete, even if it is only to check in when entering practice field. "How's it going?" "Are you having fun?" "Good practice today, you worked hard. Keep it up." Take a legitimate interest in them and what they are doing.

ADHD's Three R's

Practice and training sessions are essentially learning opportunities. And ADDers learn differently than non-ADDers learn. Generally speaking, ADDers respond best to "hands on", one to one teaching sessions with someone whose approach is closer to a mentor or master craftsman and less of a lecturer. ADDers learn from being shown how to do something rather than being told what to do.

This learning style is very much a traditional craft/apprentice experiential learning process. It relies heavily on a personal relationship of trust and mutual respect between coach and athlete. It is also the learning process that transferred knowledge and skills from one generation to another through much of mankind's existence. It is the opposite of what goes on in education today, where 30+ students may be jammed into a single classroom with the teacher lecturing from a book, unable to give every student the 1 on 1 attention that many of them, ADHD in particular, need to succeed.

Routine

Because of the distractibility issues with ADHD athletes the first key for getting the most out of practice is to have a structured environment. To the best of your ability have practices at the same time and same place during the week.

This is not to say every practice is identical. However the more routine practice or training is, the less lost, non-productive down time you and your team will experience. When routine is changed, ADDers become anxious and our sensory antennas go into active mode. We become more easily distracted and reactive to the environment around us. Unannounced or unexpected changes in routine can quickly escalate into arguments, shoving matches, and physical confrontations that take time and energy away from practice or training.

Routine is also placing athletes in competitive situations so the ADHD affected athlete becomes relaxed and confident in that situation. Routines can be infinitely chaotic and fluid or simply repetitive. The objective is to develop a sense of comfort and reduce anxiety in the athlete. When this occurs, the ADHD affected athlete begins to develop his/her abilities. They become less aware of the change around them and begin to focus on the training regimen or competition at hand, instead of being anxious about new situations.

Ritual

Rituals can be the collective acts the members of a team or club shares with one another. Some of these rituals are passed down from season to season irrespective of the athletes or the coaches. Other rituals exist for a single season.

Team rituals provide several benefits to ADHD athletes. The first is a public acceptance as a full member by the team or club. Given many ADHD athletes have often been emotionally scarred by a lifetime of being told we don't focus, don't belong, or to belong we need to change our behavior; a simple ritual such as a team huddling before a game or second half can have a tremendously positive effect. This could be the first time that the ADHD affected athlete has been accepted onto a team as a full member. The power of this can't be emphasized enough.

But rituals also provide individual structure for ADDers. For example each member of the Obukan Kendo club begins and ends each training session by bowing as they enter and leave their dojo. The members also sit together in a line and briefly meditate before each session to clear their minds of any distractions. This is done consciously with a strong emphasis on correct breathing technique. The members also bow to the senior instructor at the conclusion of each training session, thanking him for teaching them kendo. Every member understands that once training has started, they will be respectful and helpful to one another by trying to improve to the best of their ability.

During a competition or game, rituals return individual athletes to a settled place in their mind. Common examples are the shouted "Break!" before a team goes out onto a court or the huddle during a football game.

Ideally rituals will provide a mechanism for individual athletes to return their focus to "now" by clearing the consciousness of past and future distractions.

Relaxation

The objective of the three R's is for the athlete to become relaxed, focus on the right things at the right time and operate in "the zone". This is easier said than done.

There are several requirements to enter and remain in the zone. These include being competent at a particular sport. Such competence requires a number of years to develop.

Relaxation requires that someone be competent and confident in his or her actions. This requires a fundamental level of expertise in the sport or technique. It also requires that the athlete not be afraid to fail.

Keys to Training

Limit Distractions

Limit distractions at practice. This includes parents, girlfriends, boyfriends, photographers, other teams, etc. If you let distractions occur, every ADHD athlete on the team will be focusing on the difference from last practice, not what is actually going on in this practice.

Sometimes this isn't possible or practical to limit distractions. For example, if you have to share fields or gym time with another team. Or if a parent stops by to watch their child practice, it is difficult to ask them to leave, however much you might want to. Nonetheless, make every effort to foster a routine during practice or training.

Keep in mind the process is easier if this approach is implemented from the beginning of the season rather than trying to implement it later on. Do not single out the reason for the rule as "Mad Max is ADHD and if anyone shows up he won't have a good practice". Simply say you would prefer to have a minimum of distractions during practices. It has been my experience that virtually everyone will respect your wishes.

Write A Plan For Each Practice

The practice plan is just as much for the athletes as the coach. Your plan doesn't have to be minutely detailed. Listing activities and time to the nearest few minutes can serve the purpose of helping to structure your practice. A chalkboard or white board on the gym or locker room wall is ideal for sharing the plan with your team. A clipboard on the soccer or football field will work if it is shared with the team at the beginning of practice.

Remember ADDers have difficulty following only verbal instructions, particularly when there are sequential steps involved. So writing it down and posting it works to their advantage as visual learners. It also works to your advantage in moving the practice along with minimal interruptions.

A coach with a plan simply gets more done in practice than one who "wings it". Losing five minutes of training time per practice over an 11-week football season (1 September to 15 November) is over four and a half hours (25 minutes per week times 11 weeks = 275 minutes) of lost time. And this doesn't even address the increased opportunity to forget something you wanted to cover.

Once practice has started and you have finished one phase, quickly review with all athletes what activity they will be moving to next and have a group physical activity or event separating practice phase. "Okay guys on my whistle you're going to shoot free throws for the next 10 minutes. But before we get started I want you to sprint to the other end of the court and then to the foul lines. Any questions?" Tweet.

Another approach is to turn the schedule completely over to a "time keeper". One team I know of assigned their equipment manager or sometimes an injured player to keep track of practice with a stopwatch and sound a portable signal horn at the appropriate time, which also gave each coach time to quickly finish up what they were working on before starting up the next drill session.

Even if you know exactly what you are going to do in practice and have won the last five consecutive Indiana state high school basketball championships, have a written plan.

John Wooden writes he not only had a written plan for each practice, but he made certain each one of his coaches had 3x5 cards that were detailed to the minute, including what, when and where equipment was needed on the practice facility that day. He routinely spent more time planning the practice than it took to run the practice. And he kept notes. "I kept notes of every minute of every hour of every practice we ever had at UCLA."[xii]

Teach Fundamentals By Doing, Not Talking

It is a given that coaches like to talk about their sport. It is also a given that athletes would rather do the sport than hear about it or watch someone else do it. And athletes, ADDers in particular, learn a sport by actually playing it, not from watching others play it or hearing a coach talk about it. Maximize the athlete's learning time with drills that athletes will actually use during competition. Avoid having multiple lines of athletes waiting for you to watch them perform a particular skill or technique.

There are times coaches have to talk to individual athletes about new or different techniques. But when that "one to one" discussion is going on, what are the other team members doing? Are they working on their technique or are they standing in line, waiting and being unproductive?

Besides the lost productivity, having an ADDer stand in line waiting for a turn is simply asking for him or her to become distracted, impulsive and engage in "inappropriate physical activity" also known as a shoving match or argument. This in turn wastes more training time as the coach sorts things out.

One such example I learned from watching my high school basketball team (thank you Coach Iverson) warm up years ago was Basketball Tag. The player who is "it" chases four other players in an area roughly ¼ the size of a court. The only difference between tag and basketball tag is the players have to dribble a basketball the entire time. If "it" lost control of the basketball, he couldn't tag anyone out. If another player lost control, they automatically became "it". Every practice was started with this drill.

Another example I observed in a soccer practice was placing the 16 players in a large 4 by 4 square, each with the ball at his feet. The coach walked up and down the rows giving out individual instruction and encouragement as he shouted out which one of three moves he wanted the players to execute, "pull back", "step over", or "a feint".

Each player practiced the move quickly and without any wasted time. The coach called out the moves faster and faster requiring the player to execute the move with less time. But after a few minutes instead of calling just one move, he began to string them together, with players learning the motor skills to string the moves together also. More importantly the players began to grasp how one move helped set up the next move.

What all too typically happens in this situation is the coach will watch one or two players at a time execute the technique, while the other players are standing in a line waiting for their turn. In addition to taking eight times as long for the same number of repetitions is the inevitable distractions going on in the line, and the "trash talking" that would occur when a player with the ball misplays it.

The key here is having athletes learn skills by doing them, not trying to learn them by watching others do them. All too often a minority of players are actively participating, while the majority of players are passively watching and listening.

Cultivate "Continuous Chaos"

No one, ADHD affected or not, likes being placed in uncomfortable or unfamiliar situations. People don't know what to expect, what to do, what is coming next. The normal response is anxiety, tension, even fear. None of these responses are particularly useful for athletes. What happens to ADDers placed in unfamiliar situations is that in addition to the above responses, we are likely to become distracted, impulsive and reactive to our environment. Again this is simply the nature of the condition. One way to reduce or avoid this ADDer response is for the coach to inject many short bursts of intense, live, action throughout the practice. This includes drills that emphasize short periods of intense, _live_, competition.

Wrestling has a great drill where each wrestler is matched up against another one of roughly the same weight and are given 10, 20 or 30 seconds to gain an advantage or escape. No rest, no pacing, just a full out 100% effort for that short period. What is positive about this type of competitive drill is, in such a short period of time, even an overmatched wrestler has a chance to succeed (i.e. not get pinned) against even a superior wrestler, but only with a clearly focused, 100% effort. Those successes can quickly build an athlete's self esteem and also lets the ADDer become comfortable in chaos.

A soccer drill has two, four or six players, half offense and half defense. The offensive player has 10 seconds (or a few touches of the ball) to either get a shot off against the defender, pass to a player in a better scoring position, or the ball changes possession. This builds "Continuous Chaos" skills on both sides, it teaches defenders the key is staying in front of the offensive player to prevent the shot, while it teaches offensive players to speed things up and shoot before you lose possession.

For both sides it reinforces a sense of urgency for immediate action rather than waiting for the perfect situation. This urgency plays to the definitive behaviors of the ADHD athlete. Finally it teaches attack immediately when you get a turnover.

It is essential for the coach to keep the intensity level high and the praise flowing to everyone who is working hard. Praise for effort is one key building block for ADHD affected athletes. Remember this is someone who has spent much of his or her life being criticized for not being on task, for not getting things done right, for not checking his or her work, for not being neat or on time. But in competitive sports, effort and working to the best of your ability "right now" are rewarded, not criticized. No one can take the game or practice home to rework until it is perfect. ADHD athletes finally get to do something on the first take, rather than trying to make it perfect.

By constantly breaking sports down into smaller matches, the ability of ADDers can be brought to the forefront. Instead of stopping and starting during a thirty-minute scrimmage, with the accompanying rise and fall in focus and intensity, "Continuous Chaos" fosters complete focus and intensity for three minutes, ten times.

This approach also reinforces the situational awareness ADDers have. By repeatedly being placed in intense, competitive, live situations all athletes (ADDer and non-ADDer) become less anxious, less reactive, but more comfortable and relaxed than they would be in an environment of repetitively boring drills.

Finally, winning is unimportant in a "Continuous Chaos" practice. Intensity, initiative and effort are what are being taught.

Mental Training

In addition to developing physical skills and strength, every athlete will benefit from a mental training program. Just as a strength-training program is designed to develop different areas on an athlete's body, a mental training program is designed to develop different areas of the athlete's mind.

According to the United States Fencing Association[xiii], a good mental training program should include the following five Cardinal Skills: Relaxation & Activation, Concentration, Self-Talk, Imagery and Performance Routines. ADHD affected athletes will benefit significantly from a program that emphasizes concentration and positive self talk. These two areas severely impact the distractibility of the ADHD affected athlete.

Concentration is the ability to bring deliberate and conscious attention to one's performance at the right time, in the right way and in the right place. For the ADDer, learning these techniques should provide the greatest improvement in the least amount of time.

Drs. Heil & Zealand have developed a program focusing on five areas of concentration. The five areas can be practiced in total or individually. This plan starts with the athlete entering a state of relaxation.

Once in this relaxed state the program goes through a series of planned mental exercises designed to develop the athlete's ability to develop and maintain different types of concentration. By definition, ADDers benefit by developing their ability to tune out external and internal distractions.

The first exercise focuses the athlete's attention on identifying each sound (voices, footsteps, whistles) that would typically be heard in a competitive environment; labeling and identifying it so that it remains what is to be expected and then becomes less distracting to the athlete.

The second exercise focuses on the athlete becoming inwardly aware of their physical body, almost like trying to hear your own heart beat, while not being distracted by anything else.

The third exercise is controlling the flow of emotions and thoughts into the mind.... "the dark winged messengers of the psyche".

The fourth exercise is a series of eye focusing exercises, including developing peripheral vision, shifting focus from one object to another, and narrowing vision onto a single subject to the exclusion of everything else.

The intent of these exercises is twofold. First, develop and strengthen the athlete's ability to focus and maintain attention on what they need to focus and maintain attention on. Secondly, ease the transitions into and out of the different concentration styles required by any sport. Ideally this will result in a seamless movement into and out of the various attentional styles required in sport.

Positive Self-Talk is a key element for the ADHD affected athlete. ADDers have a databank full of experiences where they have fallen short of their own or other's expectations. And the ADDers' trial and error learning style guarantees that mistakes will be made. But a simple mistake on the field or practice can quickly send the ADDer down a memory lane full of lost and forgotten assignments, simple mistakes, lack of attention to detail, and impulsivity. These experiences often come flooding back in, triggering a tailspin in performance.

If the ADHD affected athlete is going to reach his or her potential they must learn how to break the cycle of negative reinforcement that such rejection and criticism bring.

One such tool is "thought stopping" and is used to shift from a negative focus to a positive focus. The steps would be 1-Stop, 2-Compose and 3-Refocus.

If an athlete becomes apprehensive about an upcoming race or bout ("I can't stay with this swimmer", "I lost to this guy last month. I'll lose to him again."), he or she must first stop the negative thought.

Then use a composure technique such as a deep breath, a flushing gesture with a hand, or other physical act that creates a separation between the negative thought and the positive thought.

The third step is to replace the negative thought with a positive one. "I am relaxed and confident", "I will move first at the gun", "I will shoot the first takedown". And then imagine or visualize performing just that act. Every time a negative thought occurs the athlete goes into a routine of 1-"Stop", 2-"Compose", 3-"Refocus-I will, I am".

It is important to note this also shifts an athlete's time focus from past negative experiences, "I lost" and future apprehensions "I will lose again" to the present, "I am ready, I will".

Coaching Objectives

Coaches throughout the world all share the same primary objective; that the athletes they coach maximize their abilities and reach their full potential.

For ADDers this is best accomplished by focusing on what each athlete controls, his or her effort, not their achievement. Achievement always follows effort; effort doesn't come from achievement.

Before Competition

Prepare team and individuals for games by focusing on what they can control and do. Not on what the opponent does. Remember the more structure that exists in a practice, the less likelihood for distractions.

Pre game meetings should focus on doing what was done in practice, not on winning. For individual sports, give athletes specific goals or objectives that he or she should perform during the competition. Make sure these goals are fully in his or her control.

Another point to keep in mind is that any changes to the race strategy or game plan needs to be explained in such a way that the ADDer understands. Simply telling an ADDer to support the player next to him or her may not be clear enough. Drawing what you want on a chalk/white board gives the ADDer more information. Asking him or her to repeat back what they heard you tell them is better because you can confirm whether or not you've been understood.

Just because an ADDer nods his or her head up and down, smiles and says, "No problem coach, I got it!" doesn't mean what you said has been understood.

Remember, coaches do their job during practices. Games and competitions are very much their exam, but they can't take it for the athlete. Athletes do their job during the competition; during the week they are studying for it.

During Competition

Mistakes will happen. If you want perfection do something besides coaching. John Wooden noted that the team that makes the most mistakes usually wins the game. What he meant is that mistakes are acts of commission, not omission. When your team or athletes aren't initiating the action, they are reacting to the opponent. That gives their opponent the edge.

Always be positive and remain in control of your emotions. Irrespective of how boneheaded a call is, keep it to yourself. If you get into a shouting match with the referee or other officials, you will be unable to correct the ADHD affected athlete if he or she does the same thing later.

And for practical purposes, I can count on one hand the times where I have seen an official or referee change a call. When they did change their call, it was after the coach had requested an explanation of the call, rather than suggesting the referee was blind or his parents had never been married.

Note: If you feel the game official's performance endangers your athletes, then pull them off the court, field, or match and take the disqualification. There isn't a sporting event in the world worth someone being crippled or dying over. But again don't get into an argument with the officials, just protect your athletes.

Keep a notebook. No one remembers everything that happens in a game. So keep notes of things as they occur during the competition so you can correct them in the next training or practice. If you have an assistant coach available, have them keep the notes. Another issue here is video taping competitions to later show athletes what they did or didn't do during the competition.

ADDers do not process verbal instructions well. We process visual commands, signals and 1v1 talks where people look us in the face. So passionately yelling verbal instructions across the field, court, mat or pool at an ADDer will usually only result in a sore throat. It likely will not result in a significant change in the competition. Keep any input you want to give during a competition to a minimum. When you do give input during competitions, hand signals or gestures may work better than verbal instruction.

If you pull someone out of the game to correct or change something, talk quietly with him or her as they come out. Show that you value them and their contribution to the team. Ask them what they think they should have done in that instance, make sure you are both on the same page with any changes and put them back in the game when it's appropriate. Glaring at him or her, and relegation to the end of the bench achieves little, except to nurture ill will and fear. John Wooden always felt that simply being "benched" was sufficient to make his point without showing anger toward a player.

It's a game and games are fun!

After Competition

Talk little, but when you do, praise personal effort and competitive action, the attempt to win and not the winning. People do not control winning or losing, they control their efforts toward winning and losing. Give out as much legitimate praise as you can. Give examples of specific individual efforts.

Tell each of your athletes what they did well, not what they did poorly. Reinforce what they did well so they want to do it again next time. Deal with the poor performance issues at the next training session.

Ask each athlete you personally coach if they are physically okay.

Make sure you look at your notes before you write the next practice plan. Where did you as a coach let the athletes down? What didn't you prepare them for? Did they fail to do something you thought had been covered?

The Off Season

The most difficult task for an ADHD athlete can be developing and executing an "off season" training regimen. It is relatively easy to maintain a high level of commitment during the season with the imposed structure of practices, games and the stimulation of teammates.

But the "off season" is when the organizational and follow through issues have the greatest opportunity to affect ADHD athletes. This is particularly true in sports with "off" seasons traditionally employing extensive and repetitive "off season" work such swimming, distance running, and with extensive weight training programs designed to build size and strength; such as throwing events or football.

What may seem to be simple tasks to the unaffected can paralyze the ADHD affected athlete. Particularly difficult is starting a multi step program. Critical to the success of the "off season" is immediately getting the athlete into a routine.

Even when ADHD athletes do make it to the pool, track or weight room for training sessions, it is likely they can become distracted and struggle to finish the training session.

To avoid, or limit the effect of these behaviors, the coach should consider the following.

Goal Setting Keys

One of the more challenging but also rewarding tasks faced by coaches and ADHD affected athletes is effective goal setting. Performing sequential, multi-step tasks is a struggle for the ADHD affected. It flies in the face of ADDer reality. So teaching ADDers how completing small jobs leads to a big success is a challenge; but it is an essential skill if ADHD affected athletes are to reach their full potential. The greatest gift anyone can give an ADDer is teaching him or her how to create and reach his or her goals. Goal setting is building skills and abilities on a step-by-step process.

There are certain principles that must be recognized.

Focus On the Performance, Not the Outcome

ADDers live in the stimulating reality of now. We don't do a good job of planning for the future nor learning from the past. Unfortunately, this doesn't do a lot of good for our long-term improvement as an athlete. So focusing on performance, or what we are doing now is key. It isn't about winning a gold medal in the Olympics; it is about doing another set on the bench press today.

Set Challenging and Attainable Goals

At the beginning of any program emphasize the attainable. If the ADDer doesn't experience success early on, it will likely be seen as boring, dull, and/or not stimulating. And if anything we are doing is boring, dull or not stimulating there is a high likelihood we will be pulled off onto something that is.

Be Positive Describing Specific Goals

Goals need to be described as what the athlete will do, not what they won't do or will stop doing. "I will make every training session," versus "I will not miss any training session." Or "I will keep my body between my opponent and the basket" and not "I will not let my opponent drive past me."

Document the Goals

Write the goals down, sign them, and post them. Also, make and keep copies. Written goals don't change, can't be forgotten or misunderstood. The signature shows everyone understands and is committed to the goals. Posting provides a visual cue or reminder to the athlete of what commitments were made to you and what his or her goals are. The athlete needs to post these goals in a visible place...on a wall, bathroom mirror, door. If they are in a file or binder they are "out of sight, out of mind".

Jointly Build a Plan

Once the goals are established, jointly construct a training plan with clearly measurable objectives to reach those goals. Simply throwing a completed plan on the desk and expecting the ADDer to follow it is unlikely to produce the needed results. As stated earlier, goal setting is the process of putting down bricks to build one wall. The athlete then builds more walls, and finally puts a roof on the house. So have a plan to turn short-term goals into intermediate goals, and long-term goals. Particular attention needs to be paid to the logistics of the plan. Where, when, who, and how will training occur?

One suggestion here is to assign a training partner or partners. It is always easier to get going and follow through with a partner or group than by yourself.

Also, try to pair up an ADDer with a non-Adder. Having two ADDers work drills together can escalate fairly quickly into confrontation or plummet just as quickly into procrastination.

Set up an initial training schedule for the athletes to work together on, and get a commitment that if they need to change the schedule, they all need to agree before the schedule is changed.

Maintain Regular Communication

It is incumbent on the coach to routinely follow up with the athletes. How are they doing? Are they having problems with any part of the off-season? Are they making progress toward their goals?

If you are a teacher in the athlete's school, make time to talk with him or her in the hallway, gym, lunchroom or wherever.

Find out how he or she is doing and reinforce their commitments to themselves and the team, not to you. "How are the sessions going?" "Anything I can help you with?" Make yourself available to watch him or her and his or her partner work out.

Being positive can't be over-emphasized.

Adjust the Plan As Necessary

It is critical for the coach and athlete to routinely communicate with one another. The athlete receives encouragement and reinforcement for the plan. The coach verifies progress is being made.

Be ready to change the plan. What happens if the athlete is injured? Can she do the same strength development program? What would have to be changed about it?

Or what would happen if a 6'3" basketball player grows six inches in a school year? What does this do to the goals he set out for himself? And incidentally, this is exactly what happened to David Robinson in his first year at the Naval Academy.

Perspective: No one wins all the time and no one loses all the time. The point of goal setting is to increase the athlete's chance of reaching his or her full potential. Set goals and do your best to reach them. But realize there are an infinite number of outcomes possible in someone's life, and most of them are beyond that person's ability to control directly. Be ready for any one of those outcomes, knowing you did your best at the time.

Unfortunately we seem to be so consumed with being "#1" or "World Champion" that we sometimes forget only one person can be "#1". If we measure success by being wealthy, then only Bill Gates is successful. If we measure athletic success with an Olympic Gold medal, then the person who won the silver medal is a loser.

Parenting the ADHD Affected Athlete

Both of my sons are ADHD affected. By 10th grade one had "retired" from organized sports completely, in large part because his coaches felt he had a "bad attitude". He didn't listen to them when they were talking, didn't do what he was told to do in games and could be disruptive (talking) when he wasn't actually playing.

His younger brother's experience was different in the beginning. During middle school (6th & 7th grade) his basketball coach coached "up tempo" style. They ran a fast break offense and defended with a full court press for the entire game, substitutions were "liberal". That team qualified for the National AAU tournament twice.

After two years (8th grade) a new coach adopted a more structured approach utilizing set plays and a zone defense. The emphasis changed to control and risk avoidance. And seemingly overnight our son developed the same "bad attitude" as his brother. My wife and I were told he didn't listen when the coach was lecturing the team, didn't do what he was told to do in games and was disruptive (talking) during practices and games. And yet his soccer coaches (both club and school) considered him extremely easy to coach and positive on the soccer field. And he was the same person around the house.

The only thing that had really changed was the particular style of play the basketball coach adopted and subsequently how that coach responded to him.

What does this mean for the parents of an ADHD affected athlete? As with anyone, sports participation can be a rewarding experience for the ADHD affected. Or it can be an experience of frustration, dread and disappointment. Sports offer ADDers a sense of accomplishment, personal responsibility, self-esteem, routine and fun. Sports also require the ADDer to structure his or her life.

But perhaps the biggest reward for the largest number of ADDers comes from interacting with people (teammates, officials, fans, competitors, siblings and, most importantly, coaches and parents) rather than in any athletic achievement.

The risk of frustration, dread and disappointment comes from continuing to experience a sense of failure from not playing, coupled with receiving a sense of disappointment from parents. Remember playing time, "success", and others opinions are not controlled by the athlete. Athletes only control one thing, their personal effort.

John Wooden, who coached ten NCAA championship teams while he was the UCLA basketball coach, defines athletic success not in terms of wins, losses or athletic achievement, but in terms of effort. Anyone working to the best of their ability, giving a full out 100% effort is successful. There is nothing more anyone can do than give a 100% effort.

The following are some suggestions for the parents of the ADHD affected athlete. They aren't a promise of success, but based on my family's personal experiences they offer the greatest opportunity for success.

Get a Full Physical

Before your son or daughter joins any organized athletic club or team ensure they receive a full physical. This is likely a requirement for anyone participating in sports today. But I put it at the top of my list to emphasize how important it is. It doesn't matter if the team, league or school requires it or not. It is simply prudent to do, particularly with anyone who might be on medication.

Accept the Situation

I know this is easier said than done, but if your ADHD affected son or daughter wants to play sports, and is physically approved by a doctor, I would hope you let them compete to the best of their ability. It might be one of the few times in their lives where he or she will be encouraged to run and jump as fast, as far and as loudly as they can.

Get a Commitment

One of the defining behaviors of ADHD is not finishing things. This includes schoolwork, homework, chores, and sometimes sports seasons. One of the first things you need to establish is a commitment for the season. And it doesn't matter how little he or she is playing. Once on a team, finish the season including practices or training sessions.

Accountability

One of my biggest concerns about sports is the "wink and a nod" some athletes receive from people that should know better. Just because someone is on an athletic team doesn't excuse bad manners, failing grades, a dirty room or a surly attitude.

Praise Personal Effort

One of America's societal standards is intolerance for mistakes or failures of any kind. I personally agree with such intolerance for building nuclear reactors or landing a 737 that I am flying on. But intolerance of athletic mistakes destroys athletes, because the only way not to make a mistake is not to try.

And therein lies a problem for athletes.

Criticizing competitive results, which are beyond the athlete's control, leads any athlete to passivity and mistake avoidance rather than giving 100% effort. This fear shows up as not swinging at a close pitch, hoping rather that the umpire calls it a ball.

But this passivity and mistake avoidance robs ADDers of more. First of all, ADDers have likely experienced more than their share of criticism. It simply comes with the condition.

Further, because ADDers are likely to be experiential learners (learning by experience rather than lectures) making mistakes is crucial to learning a skill. And to become proficient at anything, it is absolutely crucial that ADDers be allowed to make more mistakes.

The only thing any athlete really controls is personal effort. This is true at 4th grade or in the Olympics. So take the opportunity to recognize and praise legitimate hard work rather than criticizing the results.

Success requires courage and effort. Failure requires fear and passivity.

Research the Coach

Along with the parents, the coach is the most important factor in athletics being a positive or negative experience. As a parent, find out about the coach before the season starts. Talk to other parents, players from last season, or watch him or her during competition the previous season. Does the coach write a plan for each practice or do they just show up and "wing it"? Does the coach have a license or similar qualification? This isn't necessarily a critical issue, but I think it does indicate a certain level of commitment by the coach to his or her coaching.

Does the coach belong to a professional organization? One such organization is the Positive Coaching Alliance (PCA). PCA is a national body of coaches who have adopted an approach that emphasizes sports as a positive learning experience for athletes and a teaching opportunity for coaches. The emphasis is on providing positive feedback and skills to athletes, not on simply winning games.

Support the Coach

One of the biggest frustrations any youth coach has is a parent telling athletes to do the opposite of what the coach is saying. A basketball coach may want the player to pass the ball inside. But the parent screams out "Shoot the ball, you're open." This puts the athlete in a no win situation. If he shoots the coach pulls him from the game. If he doesn't shoot, he faces the inevitable parental grilling of "Why didn't you shoot the ball when you were open?" Let the coach be the coach.

Tell the Coach

I suggest you, your son or daughter tell the coach about ADHD, if for no other reason than to be honest. The coaches I know are all sincerely interested in helping their athletes succeed. Sometimes maybe not with the best of intentions, but not one of them want to see their athletes fail. If they are unaware of the situation they simply cannot do the best for their athlete. Were the situation reversed would you want to have the information? And if the coach is unfamiliar with ADHD, share what you can.

Recognize and Nurture ADHD's Gifts

Being easily distracted also means being fully aware of the environment around you. Impulsivity also means easily choosing a course of action. Hyperactivity also shows a tendency toward activity. What coach wants a player to be unaware, indecisive and inactive? Sports participation can teach ADDers how to utilize these gifts more effectively.

Finally, to the best of your ability, resist the urge to nag about what wasn't done. The past is past and irretrievable. While it might make you feel better, it is a waste of good air for getting results.

Drugs and Athletic Performance

This is an area of constant change and conflicting societal goals. The primary conflict is between the conflicting goals of legislative bodies (elected lawmakers at the national and state governments) and various athletic governing bodies (International Olympic Committee, NCAA and NAIA) regarding performance-enhancing drugs.

For example, the NAIA presently has no drug testing policy while Division I NCAA schools routinely test year round for any number of substances, including steroids. Yet within the NCAA different levels of testing exist. While D I schedules and testing are extensive, D III programs have less strict testing schedules, though the same drugs are banned for all divisions.

Some organizations have simply adopted IOC standards, which prohibit certain medications. An athlete who tests positive for any of these banned medications is disqualified and may suffer multiple year or even lifetime expulsion from competition.

This lack of a uniform standard contributes to a number of potential problems for those

ADHD affected athletes who are also students or who have jobs and careers where such medications allows them to earn a living.

On the one hand an athlete's use of physician prescribed medications for a recognized disorder is protected under U.S. Federal law including the Federal Department of Education and Americans with Disabilities Act. Yet if these athletes are tested and found with legally prescribed medications in their systems, they may be stripped of their athletic eligibility and any awards they may have won.

Generally speaking, as athletes move to higher levels of athletic competition, they become subject to increasingly stricter rules regarding medications, performance enhancing drugs and testing.

The medications most often associated with controlling attentional disorders are primarily amphetamine-based psycho stimulants (Ritalin, Adderall, Dexedrine) and are prohibited in competition by the IOC, USOC, and NCAA.

What "edge" does Ritalin provide to an athlete that makes it a banned substance for sports? In the words of the U.S. Olympic fencing organization "the primary goal for using medicines is to boost performance in the classroom environment by improving concentration and enhancing learning. It is for those very same reasons that these stimulants are beneficial to the athlete when training and competing in sport."[xiv]

That stimulant medications provide the user with increased ability to concentrate and focus shouldn't be a big surprise since this is precisely the reason these medications are prescribed to ADHD affected individuals in the first place. ADDers take medication to reduce the effect of a deficit in attentional behaviors. This increased ability to focus allows ADDers to function "normally" in society.

It is not to increase the ability to concentrate and focus to "unfair" levels or even raise them above "normal" levels enjoyed by the rest of society. They are used simply to bring the ADHD affected to "normal" levels.

That these medications enhance concentration and focus is unarguable, since that is their purpose. In that they help the ADHD affected athlete focus more clearly on learning skills, techniques, building muscle memory and conditioning, it is reasonable to conclude they help the training sessions for any sport.

Increased concentration and focus are obvious advantages when competing in "narrow internal focus" or low chaos sports such as distance running, diving, gymnastics, or shooting events. These sports reward athletes with the ability to maintain an intense singular focus on a particular task or routine, to the exclusion of everything else going on around them.

But is such increased concentration and focus an advantage when competing in all sports? Does it provide an advantage in "broad external focus", or "Continuous Chaos" sports such as boxing, soccer or ice hockey? Based on an anecdotal conversation I suspect it might even be a disadvantage.

My youngest son was diagnosed with ADHD at the beginning of high school and began taking medication (Adderall) immediately to help with his academic focus and attention. Typically the medication would "wear off" by afternoon practice time (3:00PM to 4:30PM). The one game he played while medicated was, for lack of a better term, "bloody awful". He lacked creativity, pace, or any sense of awareness as to where the game or ball were going. When I asked him about his play after the game, he told me that it was as if he couldn't shift his mind out of what it was doing. He felt as if he were 'stuck on a railroad track'. He simply couldn't "see" what was going to happen next on the field nor could he impact the game in anyway.

I recognize the inherent unreliability of such single data points. But the change in his style of play was so noticeable that several people commented on it. Since then he has played every game without medication, which is not to say he always played well. But never again did he experience the sense of being stuck on a railroad track.

If stimulant medications always provide an advantage, irrespective of the sport or event, then the athletes with the strongest concentration and learning skills should dominate every IOC sport, since it is a banned substance for every IOC sport. Yet I fail to see teams or individuals with "improved concentration and enhanced learning" abilities dominate in high chaos sports such as soccer, hockey, wrestling or boxing.

Prohibiting ADHD affected athletes from using stimulant medications because of the "edge" or performance enhancements it provides is either asking him or her to fail classes, with resultant lowered career earnings expectations for the rest of his or her life. Or it is asking the athlete to give up athletics in sports that the use of such medications may actually be a hindrance rather than an advantage.

In the United States the NCAA allows a "waiver" for ADHD affected athletes using amphetamine based medications. Each waiver must have comments from a physician establishing the medical justification including a medical history of the athlete. In Canada, the Canadian Centre for Ethics in Sport (CCES) adopted the 2004 World Anti-Doping Agency (WADA) Program. This includes lists of substances prohibited during competition and training. Ritalin, Dexedrine and Adderall are all considered S1 category drugs, which are prohibited without exception during competition, but are permitted during training. As such, students may continue to take medications during the "off season" in an academic year. Depending on how long the substance stays in an athlete's system, they have the opportunity to continue classes and compete during the academic year.

I strongly encourage coaches, doctors, parents and athletes to contact their governing bodies to determine the most current policies. All parties must remain aware of changes in this ongoing area of sports competition.

Legal Rights

Legal rights vary with country and state. In the United States those ADHD affected students who are diagnosed by appropriate medical authority are legally entitled to an Individualized Education Plan (IEP) or 504 plan if an educational impact can be shown. The IEP or 504 may include such modifications or accommodations as extended time on tests, note takers etc. And these accommodations can follow the student into university, or they may begin in university.

Because this is such a developing area of law, I simply encourage any coach or athlete to become informed of both the policy of their athletic organization and their local legislation. I would also encourage you to become active in helping others understand some of the "catch-22" situations confronting athletes on medication.

Sports for ADHD Affected Athletes

"Continuous Chaos" sports are sports where athletes continuously experience and react to an almost infinite set of events or conditions during the competition. Successful athletes in such sports must have the ability to operate with a broad externally focused concentration style, being fully aware and reactive to what is going on, rather than intensely aware of one element of the sport. As the contest is played out, it is critical that an athletes' attention move seamlessly into and out of the concentration styles. Shooting free throws is a narrow, internally focused task, while running a full court press rewards a broad externally focused concentration style.

"Continuous Chaos" sports include (but certainly aren't limited to) wrestling, boxing, soccer, martial arts and hockey. In each of these sports an athlete competes continuously without breaks or interruptions from the coach or play callers. Almost anything can happen...competitors are located throughout the playing area (right, left, ahead, or behind), and though plays occur close to goals, the overall action happens randomly throughout the playing area.

In American football, the large majority of play occurs in the middle of the field, between the 20-yard lines. This is easily verified by simply looking at a field at the end of a season. The center of it is shows a great deal of wear and tear. But looking at a soccer field (roughly the same size) at season end shows a much more uniform usage pattern. The area immediately in front of the goal shows wear and tear, but the rest of the fields tend to be in very good shape. The same can be said of ice hockey rinks where the entire surface is used equally, rather than just part of the surface.

In "Continuous Chaos" events there is a high degree of unpredictability. To play them well an athlete needs to continuously react and be aware of the entire surface throughout the contest. The "performance enhancement" provided by stimulants medications in such competitions is likely less effective than for discrete, low chaos sports which tend to be dominated by stop and go action, considerable input from coaches, and any number of routine set plays. Individual discrete, low chaos sports include diving, gymnastics, golf, swimming, and distance running (with the exception of the steeple chase and cross country). All of these sports are highly controlled, have little opportunity for chaos and emphasize perfection of technique over spontaneity.

For example, two swimmers in adjacent lanes have little ability to experience "Continuous Chaos". The swimmer with the best form (perfection of technique), cardiovascular system efficiency (repetitive distance work during training) and internal stroke rhythm will win the race.

Just as tall athletes have a higher likelihood of success in basketball and volleyball than they would have as a jockey, ADHD affected athletes have a higher likelihood of success in "Continuous Chaos" sports.

This is not to say that an ADHD affected athlete can't succeed in low chaos sports anymore than Mugsy Bogue, at 5'5", couldn't play in the NBA. Obviously he did. But for every NBA player who is shorter than 5'5", there are probably twenty who are taller than seven foot. The characteristics of the ADHD affected brain lend itself to sports with the following characteristics.

Continuous Action

Many sports, even at the professional level consist of considerable inactivity for many of the athletes. Two examples are American football and baseball/softball. A large part of these games, from when it starts to when it ends, can best be described as people waiting for the next play.

Continuous action games or sports include ice hockey, soccer, lacrosse and water polo. The one thing these sports all have in common is the game flows continuously, almost without interruption. Individual sports include the combative sports, wrestling, boxing, and martial arts, plus the racing events cycling, skating, and skiing. Substitutions in soccer occur, but at high levels can be limited to three or four in a game. They also occur continuously, without a great deal of stopping and standing. Hockey in particular can be a wonderful sport for ADDers to play since even substitutions (line changes) are made "on the fly".

Excitement

If you haven't figured out by now that ADDers crave excitement and stimulation, then please go back and read through the first part of the book again. Things have to occur on the court or field. A baseball game in the 12th inning where both pitchers are throwing no hit shut outs might be exciting for many people. But for ADDers it is more akin to watching paint flake off a building. I suspect for many of us it could be physically painful to watch. It is almost cruel and unusual punishment. At the same time, facing a fastball pitcher who throws inside can be wonderfully stimulating.

High Chaos

This is the sum of possible actions that can occur on a field, court, mat or rink. Some sports have such repetitive activity that everyone knows exactly what the opponents will do, running track for example provides little chaos (the exception being the steeple chase). The other events though consist of people running in their individual lanes for the most part and simply seeing who is faster. Admittedly for longer events, the lanes go away, but the sports remain low chaos.

Typically the ADHD athlete is interested in excitement, action and having to depend on his or her sense of awareness. Wrestling is a fabulous example of this type of sport. Even though wrestlers are limited to a twenty-five foot diameter circle to wrestle in, the direct competition with an opponent gives a huge element of chaos for both competitors.

Limited "match coaching"

Some sporting events have become agonizing exercises in the coaches' ability to counter one another's moves and counter-moves during the contest. Unfortunately, for the author anyway, the contest ends up being between the two coaches rather than a sporting event played by athletes. The traditional American sports of football and basketball are clear examples of this tendency. ADDers do not operate well in such an environment. The best sports for ADDers are those where the coach does his or her work during the week by preparing the team or individual athletes and then lets them play once the match starts.

This is not to say the coach doesn't give input during the contest. That wouldn't be a responsible approach for any coach to take. But realize once the match begins, the coach's job is largely over. The coach can make corrections or suggestions, but wholesale changes are unlikely.

High Coach to Athlete Ratio

Because of their typical learning style, ADDers are coach intensive. Having a positive, personal, relationship with a coach is critical for an ADDers' success. Remember the ADHD athlete responds best to a coach who shares his or her experience with the athlete; where the athlete is shown and guided in how to do things rather than being told how to along with 15 other players being told the same thing.

Never Being "out of it"

In most team sports (basketball, football, soccer, hockey) it is possible for the game to be over before the second half of the game starts. We've all seen the 35-zip half time football score or the 7-0 halftime soccer score. For all intents and purposes these games are decided. There is little excitement, drama or interest.

If you are suddenly thinking of one of the famous "comebacks", where a team has made up one of these half-time scores, it is only because they occur so seldom that they are memorable.

In sports such as wrestling, boxing, baseball, there is the chance for an upset right to the end of the game. Or as Yogi Berra so eloquently stated "It ain't over till it's over."

To this day I remember a university wrestling match where I was ahead 8-0 going into the final 15 seconds. I made a mistake and ended up being pinned by my opponent who didn't realize he had lost. What I learned from that match is that in some sports, it really isn't over till it's over. There is always the chance for a knockout punch, a surprise fall, a string of hits, fielding errors or a dropped baton.

Limited Off-season Work

Hopefully we've dispelled the belief that ADHD athletes are lazy and unmotivated. But off-season training programs, having little to do specifically with the sport, can be a struggle for us unless it is structured or exciting. Simply doing repetitions without the intensity of competition or without a training partner(s) can easily slide into boredom for the ADHD affected athlete.

Head to Head Competition

ADHD affected athletes enjoy competing against someone, rather than for distance, time or height. Most likely because of the stimulation such head to head competitions provide to the competitors.

Broad External Focus

ADHD affected athletes attention is focused
outwardly on the environment surrounding
them, rather than inwardly on a specific task.
Where the high jumper, diver, or gymnast is
rewarded for being inwardly focused on
performing a discrete act with perfection, the
ADDer is rewarded for performing a variety of
techniques in a constantly changing
environment. Perfection in such sports may be
desired, but not at the cost of speed of
response.

The Sports

Always keep in mind that the variable with the greatest affect on the success of an ADHD affected athlete is the coach, particulary in how he or she deals with people. The following is a brief section on specific sports for ADDers. This list is not all-inclusive nor is it exclusive. My sincere apologies to the coaches of sports I missed.

Baseball

Many people believe baseball is a poor sport for the ADHD affected athlete. And being completely honest, it is not an ADDer friendly sport. It is not a high excitement, continuous action sport. Much of the game for players consists of waiting for the batter to put the ball in play. At any one time eight of the eighteen players actually playing "in the game" are most likely sitting in the dugout, waiting for their turn at bat or waiting to go back into the field.

Still, I believe the issue is more one of where the ADDer has traditionally been placed by a coach rather than the sport itself.

In a classic "catch 22" scenario, where will a coach most likely play someone who isn't "paying attention" or seems bored with the game? The coach will position that player where the least amount of action occurs. In baseball or softball that is usually right field.

Yet, because nothing happens in right field the ADDer becomes even less interested in the game and the sport in general.

At the risk of sounding more than a little heretical, the ADDer may well blossom in areas of the game where the most action does occur; catcher, pitcher, or short stop. Catcher in particular can be an ADHD friendly position. It includes catching, throwing the ball back to the pitcher, foul balls, runners in scoring position, pick offs, base stealing, digging balls out of the dirt, etc. There is simply a lot going on for any catcher...even in a no hitter.

Basketball

Basketball can be a game of infinite possibilities and high chaos. Played throughout the world, it and soccer are as close as one can find to a "universal" game. The basic game can be played with as few as two players (1v1) on half of a court in a city playground, the street in front of your house, or even an alley way. It can be played with a fast, high intensity, take it to the hoop mindset such as Loyola Marymount utilized a number of years ago. They would simply run opponents off the floor with continuous attacking, liberal substitutions.

Another approach is to slow the game to a crawl with a zone defense and no shot clock. The game then becomes one of very finite possibilities and low chaos, where the coach has the ability to fully indulge any tendencies toward controlling both the athletes and game directly.

And recently, basketball games seem to be dominated more by the coach and less by players. Over coaching, particularly at the end of a close game, is all too prevalent with timeout, after timeout, after timeout, being called by coaches who want very much to win, but seemingly do not trust their players to finish the game unless the actions of every single player is controlled.

I watched the last five minutes of a NCAA tournament basketball game where one team continually fouled the other at every opportunity in an effort to win the game by having the other team miss free throws. It took the two teams over twenty actual minutes to complete those five game minutes. It seemed like it took much longer.

Free throws are narrow/internal focus tasks, which emphasize perfection of a single technique. By turning the game into a free throw shooting contest the coach is attempting to move the game from the upper left quadrant (broad/external focus) to the lower right quadrant (narrow/internal focus).

I am not saying this is right or wrong. But the bottom line to the suitability of the sport for ADHD affected athletes depends on the willingness of the coach to let players play in the upper left quadrant.

Football

I loved playing football. It paid my way through university. It is intense, chaotic and exciting to play. Rituals are numerous. For those who haven't played the game what may appear to be a very structured game is in reality eleven head to head competitions going on simultaneously.

Practice sessions usually start with the entire team being broken into various small groups; which in turn work on individual techniques. Interior linemen tend to work with one another. Receivers, quarterbacks and defensive backs tend to work with one another. Toward the end of each practice session these groups are brought together into defensive and offensive units, which "scrimmage" against one another.

But there are some drawbacks. At any one time in a football game only 1/3 of the team is actually on the field. When your team has the ball, both the defense and special teams are on the sideline. When the other team has the ball, your defense is on the field, the offense and special teams are on the sideline.

Additionally, there is a great deal of dead time in a game. Calling a play or setting up a defense takes up a large part of a football game today. Individual plays typically last less than six seconds while offenses have thirty-five seconds to call and start a play.

ADDers can be successful with football playing on offense, defense or special teams. Although special teams, and defense tend to be more reactive and chaotic, playing offense also provides an excellent opportunity. Particularly with the two-minute drill, the "run and shoot" or the "no huddle" offense where speed of play, reading coverage or reacting to defensive schemes on the fly is emphasized, over control from the sideline.

Hockey

Hockey is possibly the perfect team sport for an ADDer. It is a fast, intense, highly chaotic contest involving speed over the ice, and continuous action. Substitutions occur routinely within the flow of the game, without the coach needing to call a time out. The game is so fast there is no opportunity for a player to argue a call during play. If the player begins to argue, the play goes by him.

Impulsivity and physical aggression are encouraged, fighting is often considered good behavior, creativity with the puck is stressed, and individual effort is always respected and encouraged.

Coaches can only make adjustments where everyone can be spoken with between the periods. Each coach has one time out per game so there is little chance for direct control.

One of the more interesting rules in hockey is the "Penalty Box". When a player violates one of the major rules they receive a "time out" of two or five minutes in the penalty box. During this time their team will play "a man down". If the other team scores, the penalty is over. Or the penalty will end after two minutes. It is basically a cooling off period where the player can somewhat compose him or herself and reflect upon the error of his or her ways.

Soccer/Lacrosse

Soccer and lacrosse are both great sports for ADHD athletes. This is because they allow a great deal of individual creativity while in the framework of a team effort. Though the number of set plays in soccer is higher than in lacrosse, both have very high chaos levels.

Once the game starts, coaches exercise little control over the contest. Individual skills are emphasized, vision is emphasized, hard work and effort are well respected and perhaps because the sports are played year round, there tends to be little repetitive cardiovascular or weight training involved during the off season.

Racquet Sports

Racquet sports are great individual sports for ADDers. Continuous action, head to head, high chaos levels, and the only team on the court is a partner.

Of the racquet sports, tennis can be more difficult for ADDers to learn than badminton, racquetball, squash and handball (technically not a racquet sport, but included here for similarities to racquetball and squash.) What makes it a difficult game for ADHD athletes to learn is the emphasis on technique and form, dead time with chasing balls, and often the distractions of an outdoor sport. One key way to avoid this is to get as much one on one coaching as one can afford (it can be an expensive sport to learn) etc. However, once the fundamentals are mastered tennis is a wonderful, life long sport for ADDers.

Racquetball, badminton, squash and handball are easy to learn and are played in smaller, more intense areas....there is also less going on in the environment to grab the ADDers attention.

Wrestling

If one sport was ever specifically made for an ADDer, it is wrestling. Fast, intense, head to head, rewarding situational awareness, without worrying about teammates, balls or plays. The oldest recorded sport in history, wrestling is still taught in the same hands on, mentor/disciple relationship as it was 3,000 years ago. Wrestlers of the same weight compete against one another, though a 197 lb wrestler who is 6'3" tall might face another 197 lb wrestler who is 5'8" tall.

It is highly ritualized, practices are easily broken into short, intense sessions, but the coach has no ability to interrupt the match once it starts.

One of the more honest characteristics about wrestling is the coach doesn't pick who wrestles in matches. The wrestlers decide who wrestles first, second or third at each weight class. And this is determined on the mat, not by coaches.

Everyone involved in the sport always holds personal effort by a wrestler in high regard.

Finally, as long as a match is going on there is a chance for either wrestler to win.

Kendo & Martial Arts

Second only to wrestling as ADHD friendly, martial arts can produce a remarkable change in the life of the ADHD affected athlete. Kendo (Japanese fencing) in particular is fabulous because of the almost physical intensity and concentration between opponents, the personalized one on one teaching method of the sport and the emphasis on developing concentration, restraint and responsibility.

The Obukan Kendo handbook states the objectives of kendo are threefold:

Physical development (including agility, quickness, posture and poise).

Mental development including the power of concentration, the ability to make a decision and the determination to carry it out, and the willingness to "shoulder" the responsibility for actions.

Developing self-reliance and self-confidence by developing alertness, instant judgment in the face of danger, using common sense, and a sense of responsibility.

Another characteristic of kendo is that it is done at full speed at all times. This emphasis on speed allows the participants to simply react and be on the dojo floor.

One of the characteristics I most enjoy about kendo is the continuous action even during practice. There is no opportunity to "slack off". Everyone is either working on technique (waza), form (kata) or sparring (keiko). There is no standing around...only activity and movement.

Despite this constant action, practices are tightly controlled and ritualized by the sensei (instructor) and senior students. Poor etiquette is not tolerated.

Finally each practice or training session starts and finishes with a bow and period of meditation (mokuso).

The Wild Bunch Revisited

A lot has happened in the years since I coached the Wild Bunch. As I write this book, they are all in their twenties and spread out across the world. Some are attending universities, some are working, one is in Canada learning how to make films, and another is in Iraq with the United States Marine Corps.

One of the most rewarding events for me is running into or hearing about the players from that 4th grade YMCA team. Sometimes I'm called coach, and sometimes I'm not. But each one of them will mention their 4th grade basketball team. And it isn't the basketball they mention... it was the fun they had playing the game with the accelerator all the way to the floor.

I learned more about people, sports and life from that group than I learned before or since. Much of it is in this book. I hope you get the chance to learn half as much as I did.

Suggested Reading

The following is a list of books I recommend to anyone interested in learning more about working with ADHD affected athletes.

"WOODEN, A Lifetime of Observations and Reflections On and Off the Court", John Wooden with Steve Jamison, Contemporary Books, Chicago Illinois, 1997. (One of the greatest books ever written about how to help people become successful.)

"A Book of Five Rings", Miyamoto Musashi, Overlook Press, Woodstock, New York, 1974.

"The Unfettered Mind", Takuan Soho, Kodansha International, Tokyo, 2002.

"Change Your Brain, Change Your Life", Daniel G. Amen, M.D., Three River Press, New York, 1998.

"Complete Guide to ADHD", Thom Hartmann, Underwood Books, Grass Valley, 2000.

"Driven to Distraction", Edward M. Hallowell, M.D., John J. Ratey, M.D., Touchstone Book, New York, 1994.

"ADD in Adults", Dr. Lynn Weiss, Taylor Publishing, Dallas, Texas, 1992.

"Spiritual Dimensions of the Martial Arts", Michael Maliszewski, PhD, Charles E Tuttle Company, Rutland, Vermont & Tokyo 1996.